KEITH B. BILLY, MD AND VERA J. COLEMAN

The Survival Medicine Manual

The Ultimate Bug-in Guide for First Aid Self-Reliance in Emergencies

First edition

This book was professionally typeset on Reedsy.
Find out more at reedsy.com

To all those who strive to protect and care for others when circumstances become uncertain, this book is for you.

To the everyday heroes: parents, caregivers, first responders, and community members who step up when help is delayed or unavailable.

May this guide empower you with the knowledge, courage, and confidence to face any emergency with calm and skill.

And to the memory of those who inspired us to prepare and persevere your legacy fuels our commitment to survival and care.

Contents

Foreword

In an increasingly unpredictable world, the ability to respond effectively to medical emergencies is no longer a skill reserved for healthcare professionals. it is a vital necessity for everyone. Natural disasters, pandemics, accidents, and unforeseen crises remind us daily that professional medical help may not always be immediately available. When those moments come, knowledge and preparedness can mean the difference between life and death.

The Survival Medicine Manual is a comprehensive resource born out of decades of survival medicine experience and real-world necessity. It equips readers with clear, practical, and actionable medical knowledge that anyone can apply, whether you find yourself at home during a blackout, stranded in the wilderness, or in the middle of a disaster zone.

This guide goes beyond simple first aid. It empowers readers to take control of their health and safety by teaching how to build customized medical kits, manage common and complex injuries, prevent and treat infections, and even use natural remedies when conventional medicine is out of reach. It addresses chronic conditions, environmental hazards, dental emergencies, and much more & all with the goal of making survival medicine accessible and effective for the non-professional.

Whether you are a prepper, outdoor enthusiast, parent, or someone who simply values being ready for the unexpected, this book offers invaluable knowledge that can save lives. The calm confidence that comes from preparation is one of the greatest gifts you can give yourself and those you care about.

I commend the author for creating such a vital guide and encourage every reader to absorb, practice, and share the lessons within these pages. In a world where uncertainty is inevitable, preparedness is the ultimate form of empowerment.

— Keith B. Billy, MD

Acknowledgments

Creating The Survival Medicine Manual has been a journey fueled by a deep commitment to helping others be prepared, stay safe, and face emergencies with confidence. This book would not have been possible without the support, encouragement, and expertise of many individuals.

First and foremost, I want to thank the countless survival medicine professionals, emergency responders, and medical practitioners whose knowledge and dedication have inspired this work. Your real-world experience and tireless efforts to save lives have shaped the lessons shared here.

I am deeply grateful to my family and friends for their unwavering encouragement and patience throughout the writing process. Your belief in the importance of preparedness kept me motivated through every chapter.

Special thanks go to the readers and preppers who continuously seek to learn and improve their skills. Your passion and drive to protect your loved ones inspire me to keep providing valuable information.

Finally, I acknowledge the resilience of the human spirit and the strength and courage we all possess to survive, adapt, and thrive even in the most challenging circumstances. It is my hope this guide will empower you to face whatever comes your way with preparedness and peace of mind.

Preface

In a world that seems to grow more unpredictable with each passing year, the ability to care for ourselves and our loved ones in an emergency has become not just a convenience, but a necessity. Natural disasters, pandemics, civil unrest, and even personal emergencies like accidents or sudden health crises can strike without warning. Yet, too many people remain unprepared for such events, not knowing how to act or what to do when medical help is unavailable or delayed.

This guide is designed to give you the knowledge and skills you need to handle these situations, regardless of whether you're at home, in the wilderness, or anywhere in between. It's about being prepared for the worst while hoping for the best. It's about learning to trust your own abilities, understanding how to make the most of what's around you, and building the confidence to act when every second counts.

Through practical, easy-to-follow instructions and advice drawn from decades of survival medicine experience, you'll learn how to deal with injuries, illnesses, and medical crises on your own terms. Whether you're caring for yourself, your family, or someone else in need, this guide is an essential resource for anyone serious about survival.

Introduction

The Importance of Being Prepared for Medical Emergencies

We often hear the phrase "hope for the best, prepare for the worst," but how often do we truly prepare for the unexpected in a way that could save lives? Whether it's a natural disaster that isolates your community, an accident that leaves you far from help, or a medical emergency that requires immediate action, understanding how to provide medical care is a critical skill.

When disaster strikes, healthcare systems can become overwhelmed or inaccessible, leaving you to rely on your knowledge and the resources at hand. Being unprepared isn't just an inconvenience it can be a matter of life and death. Imagine finding yourself in a situation where medical supplies are limited, help is unavailable, and you're the only one who can make a difference.

This guide is not about replacing professional medical care but about giving you the tools and knowledge to manage until that help arrives or in the unfortunate event that it doesn't. The skills you'll learn here will empower you to take control of your health, your safety, and your family's well-being during medical emergencies. It's about ensuring that you're not just waiting for help, but actively becoming part of the solution.

Why Survival Medicine is Vital in Today's Uncertain World

We live in an age of unpredictability. Climate change has brought about more severe storms and wildfires. Global health crises like pandemics remind us that viruses and bacteria can spread faster than we can prepare. Political instability and social unrest can cause breakdowns in infrastructure, leaving us without access to food, clean water, or healthcare. Even more personal events like car accidents or household injuries can quickly escalate into emergencies when professional help is out of reach.

The reality is, disasters are not just for other people; they can happen to you, your family, and your community at any time. That's why survival medicine is no longer something that's nice to know it's essential. In today's world, being prepared isn't a luxury; it's a responsibility. By developing practical medical knowledge, you're not only increasing your chances of surviving an emergency, but you're also gaining a sense of confidence and control in a chaotic world.

How to Use This Guide for Personal and Family Preparedness

This guide is structured to be both a comprehensive resource and a practical manual that you can turn to in times of need. Each chapter provides in-depth, hands-on advice and training on essential survival medicine topics, from basic first aid to advanced field surgery techniques. As you read, you'll be guided through everything from building a robust survival medicine kit to understanding mental health in crisis situations.

In addition to individual preparedness, this book emphasizes the importance of family readiness. After all, survival medicine isn't just about taking care of yourself it's about being able to care for others when they need you the most. Whether it's your children, elderly relatives, or even pets, you'll learn how to tailor your medical approach to meet the unique needs of those around you.

Finally, you'll discover how to extend this knowledge to your broader community. As we'll see throughout this guide, true survival isn't just about individualism. It's about creating networks, sharing resources, and coming together to overcome adversity. The lessons here are designed to help you become a capable, calm, and effective first responder in your own life, your family's life, and your community's life.

Chapter 1: Building Your Survival Medicine Kit

In a survival scenario, your medical kit is your most important resource. Whether you're dealing with minor injuries or life-threatening situations, the contents of your kit could mean the difference between life and death. But what should go in your kit? What tools and supplies will you need? And how can you make sure you have everything without overpacking?

Key Components of a Basic Survival Medical Kit

Your basic survival medical kit should include the following key components:

- **Bandages, Gauze, and Adhesive Strips**: These are essential for controlling bleeding and covering wounds. Include a variety of sizes and types everything from large gauze pads for serious wounds to smaller adhesive bandages for cuts and scrapes.
- **Medications and Pain Relief**: Stock up on over-the-counter pain relievers like ibuprofen and aspirin, as well as any personal medications you may need. Don't forget medication for common ailments like allergies or nausea.
- **Antiseptics and Disinfectants**: Infections can quickly turn a minor injury into a major health crisis, especially in environments where healthcare is unavailable. Ensure your kit includes antiseptics, alcohol wipes, and other disinfecting solutions.
- **Tools: Thermometers, Scissors, Tweezers**: Thermometers help you

monitor fevers, which can indicate infection or illness. Scissors and tweezers will be invaluable for cutting gauze, bandages, or even removing splinters and foreign objects.

Advanced Kit Items: Surgical Tools and Emergency Supplies

Once you have your basic kit assembled, consider adding more advanced items, including surgical tools, chest seals, and hemostatic agents. These will be necessary if you find yourself in a situation requiring more advanced care, such as severe trauma or life-threatening bleeding.

Customizing Your Kit for Specific Needs

One size does not fit all when it comes to medical kits. You'll need to adjust your kit to meet the specific needs of yourself and your family. If you have young children, for instance, be sure to include child-sized bandages and medications. For elderly family members, consider including medications for chronic conditions or specialized equipment like blood pressure cuffs.

Pets also require specific care, so if you have animals, make sure to include medications, bandages, and other supplies for them as well.

How to Store and Maintain Your Medical Kit

The best survival medical kit is useless if you can't access it or if it's poorly maintained. Store your kit in a dry, cool place that's easy to get to in an emergency. You should also regularly check the contents to ensure that medications haven't expired, bandages are intact, and tools are in working condition.

Ensuring Your Kit is Portable

You may need to move your kit quickly in the event of an evacuation. Choose containers that are durable and lightweight but large enough to store everything you need. A well-organized backpack or duffel bag is ideal for portability and easy access.In a survival situation, a well-stocked and organized medical kit can be your lifeline. It's not just about having the right supplies it's about ensuring that those supplies are easy to access, use, and maintain. As you build your kit, remember that it needs to be both comprehensive and practical, designed with your unique needs in mind. In this section, we'll explore how to select and organize your medical kit for maximum effectiveness.

Key Components of a Basic Survival Medical Kit (Expanded)

While every medical emergency is different, there are common elements that should be present in every survival medicine kit. These items are designed to address a range of injuries, illnesses, and conditions that might arise during a disaster or emergency.

- **Bandages, Gauze, and Adhesive Strips**:When a wound occurs, stopping bleeding quickly is the top priority. Bandages, sterile gauze pads, and adhesive strips are critical for this. You should have a variety of sizes small bandages for cuts and abrasions, larger ones for deeper wounds, and gauze pads for covering larger or more severe injuries. A few rolls of cohesive bandage are also essential as they can be wrapped around limbs and joints to hold other bandages in place. In addition to these, include self-adhesive bandages, such as "butterfly closures," which are invaluable for closing up small lacerations or cuts.
- **Medications and Pain Relief**:Pain can impair your ability to focus and act during a medical emergency, so being able to manage it is important. Include pain relievers like **acetaminophen** (Tylenol), **ibuprofen** (Advil), and **aspirin**. For non-prescription anti-inflammatory medication, you may want to stock **naproxen** (Aleve). It's also wise to add medications for common ailments, such as **antihistamines** for allergies or **anti-nausea tablets**. Don't forget **prescription medications** for chronic conditions you may have (like insulin for diabetes or heart medications), and keep them in their original bottles with the doctor's prescription attached.
- **Antiseptics and Disinfectants**:Preventing infection is crucial when you're dealing with injuries in survival situations. Without proper hygiene and sanitation, a minor cut could become a life-threatening infection. In your kit, include **hydrogen peroxide** (3%), **alcohol wipes**, and **antiseptic ointments** like **Neosporin**. For cleaning large wounds, **iodine tinctures** or **betadine solution** can help disinfect the area before dressing the wound. You may also want to carry a **saline solution** for irrigating wounds or flushing out dirt and debris.

- **Tools: Thermometers, Scissors, Tweezers**:Medical tools make it easier to assess and treat injuries. **Thermometers** will help you monitor body temperature and identify fevers. **Scissors** (preferably bandage scissors, which are designed for cutting through cloth without harming the skin) are essential for cutting tape, gauze, or clothing to access injuries. **Tweezers** should be included for removing splinters, glass, or insect stingers. A **hemostat** (a type of clamp) can be useful for controlling bleeding or stabilizing a wound during the dressing process. Additionally, a **flashlight** is critical in case of power outages, especially during evening hours when visibility is poor.
- **Sterile Gloves**:Wearing gloves during medical procedures helps prevent infection and protects both you and the injured party. Pack at least two pairs of sterile, disposable gloves. If you have family members with latex allergies, opt for **nitrile gloves**, which are latex-free but still offer a high level of protection.

Advanced Kit Items: Surgical Tools and Emergency Supplies

Once you've covered the basics, consider adding more specialized items to your survival medicine kit. These tools are necessary in more extreme situations where you might need to perform more advanced care or surgery.

- **Surgical Tools**:While it's highly unlikely that you will need to perform surgery in a survival situation, having some basic surgical tools on hand can be lifesaving in extreme emergencies. This could include tools like **scalpels, surgical scissors, forceps**, and **needle holders**. These items will help if you need to cut away infected tissue or stitch up a serious wound. For suturing, you'll need **sterile sutures** and an appropriate **needle**. It's also important to have a basic knowledge of how to use these tools, which is why this guide will delve into field surgery techniques in later chapters.
- **Tourniquets and Hemostatic Agents**:A **tourniquet** can be a life-saving tool for controlling severe bleeding, especially in cases where direct

pressure isn't enough to stop hemorrhaging. These should be of high quality, such as a **CAT tourniquet**, and easy to apply. **Hemostatic agents** (e.g., **QuikClot**) help speed up clotting in deep wounds. They're often used in military and field medicine but are becoming essential for civilian kits as well. These items are crucial for controlling massive blood loss, which could otherwise be fatal within minutes.

- **Chest Seals**:If someone suffers from a gunshot wound or a stab wound to the chest, the risk of air entering the chest cavity (a pneumothorax) can collapse the lung. **Chest seals** are adhesive dressings that are used to seal the wound and prevent air from entering. These items are highly specialized but important if you're likely to be in environments where such injuries could occur.
- **Burn Care Supplies**:Burn injuries, especially in a wilderness or survival setting, are a significant concern. Include **burn dressings** or **gel** that cool and protect burn areas. You should also pack **sterile gauze** and **non-stick pads** to prevent the burned skin from sticking to the dressing. **Burn blankets** can also be useful for larger burns, as they provide cooling and prevent further damage from heat exposure.

Customizing Your Kit for Specific Needs

A good survival medical kit is personalized. Whether you have children, elderly relatives, pets, or any other special needs in your family, customizing your kit ensures that you're ready for whatever situation arises.

- **For Children**:If you have young children, you'll need to account for their size and age when preparing your kit. Stock **baby wipes**, **diapers**, and **children's medications**, such as liquid versions of pain relievers and fever reducers. Remember that children are more prone to dehydration, so **oral rehydration salts** and pediatric electrolyte solutions should also be included. Additionally, ensure that any **pediatric first aid guides** or instructions are in your kit, so you can act quickly if your child sustains an injury or illness.

- **For Elderly Relatives**:Older individuals often have unique medical needs, such as managing **chronic conditions** (diabetes, hypertension, arthritis) or cognitive issues. Make sure you have extra supplies of any medications they take regularly. **Blood pressure cuffs, glucometers** (for measuring blood sugar), and **diabetic test strips** are important for monitoring their health. Additionally, elderly individuals may be at greater risk for falls, so be sure to include **pain relief** and **muscle rubs**, as well as bandages suitable for thinner skin, which may tear more easily.
- **For Pets**:Animals need medical care too. A pet-specific first aid kit should include **bandages, wound disinfectants, antibiotic ointments**, and **sutures**. Consider carrying **flea and tick treatments** and any **medications** your pets require, especially for heartworms or motion sickness. Don't forget **pet-friendly pain relievers** (don't use human painkillers on pets), and always have a list of emergency animal hospitals or veterinarians on hand.

How to Store and Maintain Your Medical Kit

A survival medical kit does no good if it's inaccessible or in disrepair. Proper storage and maintenance are critical. Here's how you can ensure that your kit is always ready when you need it:

- **Choose the Right Container**:Opt for a durable, water-resistant container that will protect the contents from environmental factors like moisture, heat, and dirt. A **tactical backpack** or a large, waterproof **duffel bag** is ideal because it allows you to keep everything in one place and carry it easily in an emergency. You can also use clear plastic boxes with secure lids for organizing smaller items.
- **Organization is Key**:A disorganized kit is almost as bad as having no kit at all. Use **zippered pouches** or **compartmentalized cases** to group similar items together. Label each section for easy identification "Bandages," "Medications," "Tools," and so on. This will save you precious time when every second counts.

- **Regular Checks and Maintenance**:The contents of your medical kit should be checked regularly. Medications have expiration dates, bandages can become damaged, and tools can rust or break. Make it a habit to check your kit at least twice a year to ensure that everything is in working order. Make sure medications are still within their shelf life and that all supplies are complete and intact.

Ensuring Your Kit is Portable: Choosing the Right Bag and Containers

When disaster strikes, you may need to evacuate quickly. That's why portability is an important factor when choosing a container for your medical kit. A sturdy, well-designed bag should have the following features:

- **Lightweight yet durable**: You don't want to be weighed down by an overly heavy kit, but it should be made of high-quality material to withstand the rigors of rough handling.
- **Multiple compartments**: This helps you keep supplies organized and easily accessible in a crisis. Having a separate compartment for each category of supplies (bandages, tools, medications, etc.) can save time when searching for the right item.
- **Comfortable carrying straps**: If you need to carry your medical kit for long distances, padded, adjustable straps can make a huge difference in comfort.

By following these guidelines, you'll have a well-equipped, easy-to-carry, and well-maintained survival medicine kit ready for any situation. Remember, preparedness is key. The more thought and effort you put into creating your kit now, the more confidence you'll have when it's needed most.

Chapter 2: First Aid for Common Injuries and Trauma

In any emergency, injuries are inevitable. Whether you're dealing with a minor cut from a kitchen accident or a life-threatening trauma from a natural disaster, having the knowledge and supplies to treat common injuries is critical for survival. The key to effective first aid is to act quickly and calmly, following a systematic approach to address the injury, stabilize the individual, and prevent further harm. In this chapter, we will explore a wide range of injuries and trauma scenarios, providing step-by-step guidance on how to treat them in a survival setting.

Wound Care: Cleaning, Dressing, and Preventing Infection

Wound care is perhaps one of the most fundamental skills in survival medicine. Whether the wound is the result of an accident, animal bite, or a traumatic event, proper cleaning and dressing are essential to prevent infection and facilitate healing.

- **Assessing the Wound**The first step in treating any wound is assessing the severity. Is the wound superficial, or is it deep? Does it involve major blood vessels, muscles, or internal organs? Identifying the type of wound will guide your treatment plan.
- **Minor Cuts and Scrapes**: If the wound is superficial and only involves the outer layers of skin, you can typically treat it at home. Minor cuts can be cleaned with mild soap and water to remove dirt and debris.

- **Lacerations and Puncture Wounds**: Deeper lacerations or puncture wounds may involve bleeding from blood vessels. These wounds should be cleaned thoroughly to avoid infection, and in some cases, you may need to apply pressure to stop the bleeding.
- **Grazes and Abrasions**: These are superficial injuries where the skin is scraped, often leaving an area of raw tissue exposed. While not typically serious, these wounds can still become infected if not cleaned and dressed properly.
- **Cleaning the Wound**Proper cleaning is critical to avoid infection. You should always wash your hands thoroughly before touching any wound. If possible, use **sterile saline solution** to rinse the wound. If you don't have saline, use clean water, but avoid using harsh chemicals like hydrogen peroxide or alcohol, as they can damage healthy tissue and delay healing. For more severe wounds, apply **antiseptic ointment** to reduce the risk of infection.
- **Dressing the Wound**Once cleaned, the wound needs to be dressed. Use **sterile gauze** or **non-stick pads** to cover the area. Apply a **bandage** to hold the dressing in place. It's important not to wrap the bandage too tightly, as it can impede circulation. If the wound is bleeding heavily, apply direct pressure with a clean cloth or gauze to control the bleeding. In case of large or serious wounds, use **pressure bandages** to apply consistent pressure and reduce blood loss.
- **Preventing Infection**The greatest risk to any wound is infection. To prevent infection, keep the wound covered with a sterile dressing, and change the bandages daily or whenever they become wet or dirty. If the wound begins to show signs of infection (redness, swelling, increased pain, or pus), seek medical attention as soon as possible. In the absence of modern medical resources, **antibiotics** (which should be included in your survival medicine kit) can help treat infection, but these should be used with caution, as improper use can lead to resistance.

Treating Sprains, Strains, and Fractures: Splinting Techniques

Sprains, strains, and fractures are among the most common injuries in emergency situations, especially during outdoor activities or in high-stress environments. Understanding how to treat these injuries effectively is vital for minimizing pain, preventing further damage, and facilitating healing.

- **Sprains and Strains**A **sprain** involves the stretching or tearing of ligaments, while a **strain** involves damage to muscles or tendons. Both types of injuries typically occur when a joint or muscle is overexerted or subjected to unnatural movement.
- **Signs and Symptoms**: Sprains and strains often present with swelling, pain, bruising, and limited mobility. In severe cases, there may be noticeable deformity or the inability to move the joint.
- **First Aid Treatment**: The primary treatment for sprains and strains follows the **R.I.C.E. method** Rest, Ice, Compression, and Elevation.
- **Rest**: Avoid using the affected joint or muscle. Immobilize it if possible.
- **Ice**: Apply ice packs wrapped in a cloth to reduce swelling and pain. Do this for 20 minutes at a time, every hour for the first 24-48 hours.
- **Compression**: Wrap the injury with an elastic bandage to reduce swelling, but make sure it's not too tight to avoid cutting off circulation.
- **Elevation**: Raise the injured area above heart level to help reduce swelling.
- **Fractures**Fractures (broken bones) are more serious than sprains and strains. They can involve simple fractures, where the bone breaks but does not pierce the skin, or compound fractures, where the bone punctures the skin, potentially leading to severe infection.
- **Signs and Symptoms**: Fractures are often accompanied by pain, swelling, and bruising. If the bone is broken, there may be visible deformity or an unnatural angle to the limb. You may also hear a cracking sound at the moment of injury.
- **First Aid Treatment**: If you suspect a fracture, immobilize the affected limb immediately to prevent further injury. The goal is to prevent the bone from moving and causing additional damage.
- **Splinting**: A **splint** is an essential tool for immobilizing fractures. If

you don't have a commercial splint, you can make one from available materials, such as a sturdy branch or piece of wood. The splint should extend above and below the fracture site and be padded with cloth to minimize discomfort. Use **bandages or strips of cloth** to secure the splint in place, making sure not to apply pressure that would cut off circulation. The splint should allow for some movement but prevent the fractured area from moving.

- **Elevation**: Elevate the injured limb as much as possible to reduce swelling.
- **Pain Relief**: Administer pain-relieving medication, such as **ibuprofen** or **acetaminophen**, if available.

Basic Burn Care: From Minor Burns to Severe Cases

Burns can range from minor discomfort to life-threatening injuries. They can be caused by heat, chemicals, electricity, or radiation. Understanding how to treat burns quickly and effectively can minimize the damage and significantly improve recovery outcomes.

- **Types of Burns**
- **First-Degree Burns**: These affect only the outer layer of the skin (epidermis) and cause redness, pain, and mild swelling. Sunburn is a common example.
- **Second-Degree Burns**: These involve the deeper layers of the skin (dermis) and cause blisters, more severe pain, and swelling.
- **Third-Degree Burns**: These burns are the most serious and involve all layers of the skin, possibly affecting underlying tissues. There may be no pain at the burn site (due to nerve damage), but the area will appear charred or white and dry.
- **Burn First Aid**
- **First-Degree Burns**: Cool the burn by running it under cold (not ice-cold) water for at least 10 minutes. Cover the burn with a clean, non-stick dressing and apply **aloe vera gel** or **burn ointment** for pain relief.

- **Second-Degree Burns**: After cooling the burn, cover it with a sterile bandage or non-stick gauze. Do not pop any blisters, as this increases the risk of infection. If blisters break, clean the area and apply an antibiotic ointment.
- **Third-Degree Burns**: Do not attempt to remove clothing stuck to the burn or treat the area with water. Instead, cover the burn with a clean, sterile cloth or bandage to protect it from infection. Seek emergency medical care immediately.
- **General Burn Treatment Tips**Always monitor for signs of **shock**, especially in severe burns. Keep the victim warm, hydrated, and in a position that minimizes strain on their body. **Pain management** is also essential for burn patients, as burns can cause significant discomfort. In cases of serious burns, be prepared to administer **IV fluids** or other forms of advanced care, which will be covered later in the book.

How to Treat Cuts, Scrapes, and Blisters in Emergency Settings

Even minor cuts, scrapes, and blisters can become serious if not treated properly. In a survival situation where medical assistance is unavailable, these seemingly minor injuries can quickly escalate into infections or more significant health problems.

- **Cuts and Scrapes**The first step in treating cuts and scrapes is to clean the wound thoroughly. Use **sterile saline solution** or clean water to irrigate the area and remove any dirt or debris. Once cleaned, apply an **antiseptic ointment** and cover the wound with a sterile bandage to protect it from infection. For more significant cuts, you may need to apply pressure to stop the bleeding and even use a **sterile dressing** to prevent further contamination.
- **Blisters**Blisters are common, especially during physical activity or in hot environments. If a blister is small and intact, leave it alone and cover it with a bandage to protect it from further irritation. If the blister is large or painful, you can carefully drain it by sterilizing a needle and

puncturing the blister at the base. Once drained, apply an **antibiotic ointment** and cover the area with a sterile dressing.

Recognizing and Responding to Shock

Shock is a life-threatening condition that occurs when the body's organs and tissues don't receive enough blood flow. It can be caused by trauma, blood loss, severe burns, infections, or even dehydration. Recognizing the symptoms of shock early and providing immediate treatment can make the difference between life and death.

- **Signs of Shock**
- Pale, cold, and clammy skin
- Weak, rapid pulse
- Rapid breathing or shortness of breath
- Nausea or vomiting
- Confusion or disorientation
- **First Aid for Shock**The primary treatment for shock is to **restore blood flow** to vital organs and maintain the person's body temperature. To treat shock:
- **Lay the person down** with their legs elevated to help increase blood flow to the heart and brain.
- **Cover them** with a blanket or clothing to maintain body heat.
- **Keep the person calm** and ensure that they are breathing steadily.
- If the person is conscious, encourage them to drink small sips of water or an electrolyte solution to prevent dehydration.

In severe cases, shock can lead to **cardiac arrest**, requiring CPR (which we will cover later). Always seek professional medical help as soon as possible, even in a survival situation, as shock can be rapidly fatal without proper treatment.

CPR and Basic Life Support (BLS): A Vital Skill for Everyone

CPR (cardiopulmonary resuscitation) is one of the most important life-saving skills you can learn. Whether someone has suffered from a heart attack, drowning, or trauma, CPR can buy valuable time until more advanced medical care arrives.

- **How to Perform CPR**
- **Check for responsiveness**: Tap the person gently and shout, "Are you okay?" If there's no response, proceed to the next step.
- **Call for help**: If possible, have someone call emergency services while you begin CPR.
- **Chest Compressions**: Place the heel of one hand on the center of the person's chest, just below the sternum. Place your other hand on top and interlace your fingers. Push hard and fast, at a rate of 100-120 compressions per minute, allowing the chest to rise fully between compressions.
- **Rescue Breaths**: After 30 compressions, give the person 2 rescue breaths by tilting their head back, lifting the chin, and sealing your mouth over theirs. Give each breath over 1 second, making sure the chest rises.
- **Repeat**: Continue chest compressions and rescue breaths until the person starts breathing or emergency help arrives.

Conclusion of Chapter 2

As you can see, first aid for common injuries and trauma is not just about having the right supplies it's about knowing how to use those supplies effectively and acting quickly in a calm and confident manner. Every injury, no matter how small, deserves your attention. By mastering these basic first aid techniques, you'll be able to provide care to yourself, your loved ones, and even strangers, ensuring that you're ready to face any medical emergency, no matter how dire. In the next chapter, we will dive deeper into treating infections and illnesses in survival situations, equipping you with the knowledge to handle sickness when conventional medical help is unavailable.

Chapter 3: Treating Infections and Illnesses in Survival Situations

In any survival situation, whether you're stranded in the wilderness, facing a natural disaster, or dealing with a long-term crisis, one of the greatest challenges is managing infections and normally be treated with antibiotics, hospital care, or specialized treatments can quickly become life-threatening when medical help is unavailable. The knowledge and skills to effectively treat infections, manage common illnesses, and prevent diseases are critical to surviving in these situations.

This chapter will provide you with essential knowledge on how to recognize, treat, and prevent infections and illnesses during a survival situation. It covers everything from identifying common infections to managing respiratory illnesses and gastrointestinal disorders, as well as the use of natural remedies when pharmaceuticals are unavailable. The goal is to give you a comprehensive approach to keeping yourself and your loved ones healthy when modern medicine is out of reach.

Recognizing Signs of Infection and Sepsis

Infections are a leading cause of death in survival scenarios because they often go unnoticed or untreated for too long. The body's immune system can be overwhelmed, leading to **sepsis**, a potentially fatal condition in which the body's response to infection causes widespread inflammation and damage to organs.

- **Signs of Infection**The first step in dealing with infections is recognizing them early. Common signs of infection include:
- **Redness** around a wound or injury site
- **Swelling** at the site of infection
- **Heat** emanating from the wound or infected area
- **Pus or discharge** from the wound
- **Pain** or tenderness
- **Fever** (a body temperature above 100.4°F or 38°C)
- **Chills or sweating**
- **Fatigue** and malaise

Infections can range from mild to severe. The more severe the infection, the more serious the consequences. If you notice any of these signs of infection, immediate intervention is crucial to prevent it from worsening into sepsis.

- **Signs of Sepsis**Sepsis occurs when an infection spreads throughout the body, causing the immune system to attack its own tissues. This is a medical emergency that requires immediate attention. Some signs of sepsis include:
- **Rapid heart rate** (tachycardia)
- **Low blood pressure** (hypotension), which can lead to dizziness or fainting
- **Rapid breathing** (tachypnea)
- **Confusion, disorientation, or agitation**
- **Cold, clammy skin**
- **Cyanosis** (a bluish tint to the skin, especially around the lips and fingers)

If sepsis is suspected, it's important to act immediately. The best course of action is to clean and dress any wounds or infected areas, elevate the person's legs to improve circulation, and keep them warm. If you have access to antibiotics, administer them as soon as possible and seek professional medical help immediately.

How to Identify and Treat Common Infections

In a survival situation, the types of infections you might encounter will vary based on the environment, the nature of the injury or illness, and the resources available. Here, we'll discuss how to recognize and treat some of the most common types of infections that can occur in a survival setting.

- **Skin Infections**Skin infections often result from cuts, scratches, or insect bites. The two most common types are **cellulitis** and **impetigo.** Cellulitis is a deep skin infection, while impetigo is a superficial bacterial infection often caused by **Staphylococcus aureus** or **Streptococcus pyogenes**.
- **Treatment**: Begin by cleaning the wound or injury with **sterile saline solution** or clean water. Apply an **antiseptic ointment** to the infected area and cover it with sterile gauze or a bandage. If the infection worsens or spreads rapidly, it may be necessary to administer **oral antibiotics** if available (e.g., **amoxicillin** or **penicillin**). If the infection does not improve, you may need to apply a **hot compress** to the area to draw out infection and facilitate drainage.
- **Urinary Tract Infections (UTIs)**A urinary tract infection (UTI) is another common condition that can become serious if left untreated. Symptoms include painful urination, frequent urination, cloudy or foul-smelling urine, and lower abdominal pain. UTIs are especially prevalent among women in survival situations.
- **Treatment**: Hydration is key. Encourage the person to drink plenty of clean water. **Cranberry juice** has long been considered a natural remedy for UTIs, as it can help prevent the bacteria from adhering to the walls of the urinary tract. If possible, administer **antibiotics** to treat the infection. A broad-spectrum antibiotic like **ciprofloxacin** can be effective for UTIs, but if no antibiotics are available, **garlic** and **parsley** have been used in traditional medicine to help treat UTIs. Maintain proper hygiene and have the individual urinate as soon as they feel the urge.
- **Respiratory Infections**Respiratory infections, including the **common cold**, **influenza**, and **pneumonia**, are common in environments where

hygiene is poor or when the body's immune system is stressed. In a survival scenario, these infections can quickly escalate into something more serious, especially if you're in a confined space or exposed to cold weather.

- **Treatment**: For mild respiratory infections, ensure the individual rests and drinks plenty of fluids. **Steam inhalation** can help loosen mucus and ease congestion. If the person has a fever, administer fever-reducing medications like **ibuprofen** or **acetaminophen**. If pneumonia is suspected, the person will likely need antibiotics (if available), but rest and proper hydration are vital to preventing further complications. In severe cases of respiratory distress, you may need to assist with breathing techniques and monitor for signs of **hypoxia** (low oxygen levels).
- **Gastrointestinal Infections**Gastrointestinal illnesses, including food poisoning, **gastroenteritis**, and **diarrhea**, are common in survival settings, particularly when access to clean water and sanitation is limited. These infections can lead to **dehydration**, which can be life-threatening if untreated.
- **Treatment**: The primary treatment for gastrointestinal infections is hydration. Oral rehydration solutions (ORS) can replace lost fluids and electrolytes. If ORS is unavailable, a mixture of **1 liter of water**, **6 teaspoons of sugar**, and **1/2 teaspoon of salt** can be used to rehydrate the body. **Probiotics** or **activated charcoal** can help restore the balance of healthy bacteria in the gut. If diarrhea is severe and persistent, administer an **antidiarrheal medication** (such as **loperamide**) if available. Avoid solid food until symptoms improve.

Managing Respiratory Illnesses (Colds, Flu, Pneumonia)

Respiratory infections are common, especially in cold weather or when hygiene is poor. In a survival scenario, respiratory illnesses can be difficult to manage due to a lack of proper healthcare resources and the potential for rapid spread among groups of people.

- **Common Cold**The common cold is a viral infection that affects the upper respiratory tract. Symptoms include a runny or stuffy nose, sore throat, cough, mild body aches, and mild fever.
- **Treatment**: There is no cure for the common cold, but symptoms can be managed. Ensure the person gets plenty of rest and stays hydrated. **Warm saltwater gargles** can soothe a sore throat, and **hot tea** with **honey** and **ginger** can help relieve congestion. Over-the-counter **decongestants** and **pain relievers** (like ibuprofen or acetaminophen) can also help alleviate symptoms.
- **Influenza (Flu)**The flu is more severe than the common cold, with symptoms that include fever, chills, fatigue, muscle aches, and sore throat. The flu can lead to serious complications, including pneumonia, particularly in the elderly or those with weakened immune systems.
- **Treatment**: Flu symptoms can be managed with **fluids**, **rest**, and **pain relievers**. If antiviral medications like **Tamiflu** are available, they can help reduce the severity and duration of symptoms. If not, focus on supportive care, such as rest, hydration, and fever management. Keep the person isolated to prevent the spread of the virus to others.
- **Pneumonia**Pneumonia is a serious respiratory infection that affects the lungs. It can be caused by bacteria, viruses, or fungi and leads to symptoms such as cough, fever, chest pain, difficulty breathing, and fatigue. If pneumonia is not treated promptly, it can lead to severe complications, including respiratory failure.
- **Treatment**: Pneumonia requires immediate medical attention, but in a survival scenario, you can still provide critical care. Administer antibiotics (if available) and ensure the person stays warm and hydrated. You should monitor their breathing closely. If breathing becomes shallow or labored, help them into a sitting or semi-upright position to facilitate easier breathing. **Oxygen therapy** is critical in severe cases, so if you have access to supplemental oxygen, use it as necessary. Keep the patient comfortable, and seek medical help at the earliest opportunity.

Treating Digestive Disorders: Diarrhea, Vomiting, and Dehydration

Gastrointestinal illnesses are common in survival settings, particularly when food and water are scarce or contaminated. They can quickly lead to dehydration, malnutrition, and weakened immunity.

- **Diarrhea**Diarrhea can result from infections, contaminated food, or stress. It leads to rapid fluid loss, which can cause dehydration if not treated properly. Symptoms include frequent, loose stools, abdominal cramping, and sometimes fever.
- **Treatment**: The primary goal in treating diarrhea is to prevent dehydration. Oral rehydration solutions (ORS) are crucial for replacing lost fluids and electrolytes. If ORS is unavailable, make your own using water, salt, and sugar. Avoid solid foods until symptoms improve, and stick to clear liquids. In cases of severe diarrhea, **antidiarrheal medications** like **loperamide** can be used to slow the passage of stool and prevent further fluid loss.
- **Vomiting**Vomiting can be caused by a variety of factors, including infection, food poisoning, and stress. Prolonged vomiting leads to dehydration and the loss of essential electrolytes.
- **Treatment**: Rehydrate the individual with small sips of water or an electrolyte solution. **Ginger tea** can help soothe the stomach and reduce nausea. If vomiting is severe and persistent, consider using **anti-nausea medications** (if available), or try home remedies like **acupressure** on the wrist or applying a cool compress to the forehead.
- **Dehydration**Dehydration occurs when the body loses more fluids than it takes in. This condition can be exacerbated by diarrhea, vomiting, or excessive sweating.
- **Treatment**: Rehydrate the individual immediately using an oral rehydration solution (ORS). If no ORS is available, prepare a mixture of water, sugar, and salt to help restore fluid balance. Make sure the individual drinks small sips frequently rather than large amounts at once, which can worsen nausea. If dehydration becomes severe, intravenous fluids may be necessary, but this will require medical intervention.

How to Prevent and Treat Waterborne Diseases in the Wild

Waterborne diseases are a significant concern when you're in a survival situation, particularly in environments where water sources are contaminated. Pathogens like **Giardia**, **Cryptosporidium**, and **E. coli** can contaminate water, leading to gastrointestinal illnesses and dehydration.

- **Prevention**
- Always boil water for at least one minute to kill harmful pathogens.
- If boiling isn't possible, use **water purification tablets** or a **water filter** to remove contaminants.
- Avoid drinking water from stagnant or dirty sources, as they are more likely to contain harmful bacteria or parasites.
- **Treatment**If you suspect someone has a waterborne disease, ensure they stay hydrated and monitor their symptoms closely. Use **activated charcoal** to help absorb toxins in the digestive system, and if possible, administer **antibiotics** for bacterial infections. For parasitic infections like **Giardia**, medication like **metronidazole** can be effective, though it's essential to have access to these medications in a survival situation.

Managing Fever and Its Symptoms Without Modern Medicine

Fever is a common symptom of many infections and illnesses. It's the body's natural defense mechanism to fight off infection, but if left untreated, it can cause discomfort and lead to complications like **febrile seizures** in young children or **heat stroke** in extreme cases.

- **Managing Fever**To manage a fever in a survival setting, start by ensuring the person stays hydrated. Apply a **cool compress** to the forehead or back of the neck to bring their body temperature down. **Teas** made from **willow bark** or **feverfew** can help reduce fever, as these herbs contain natural compounds that act like aspirin. If the fever is high (over 104°F or 40°C), it's important to **cool the person down slowly** and monitor their condition closely.

Using Natural Remedies for Minor Ailments

When conventional medicine is not available, natural remedies can be invaluable for treating minor illnesses and ailments. Many plants, herbs, and natural substances have powerful healing properties that can support the body during times of crisis.

- **Herbal Remedies**:Herbs like **echinacea** for immune support, **peppermint** for digestion, and **lavender** for calming anxiety and promoting sleep can all be useful additions to your survival medicine kit. Always ensure that you can properly identify herbs before using them, as some plants can be toxic if misused.
- **Garlic**:Known for its antimicrobial properties, garlic can help treat a variety of infections. It can be used both topically (as a paste) and internally (as part of a tea or in food) to combat bacteria and fungi.
- **Honey**:Honey has natural **antibacterial properties** and has been used for centuries to treat wounds, burns, and throat infections. It can also be used as a natural cough suppressant.

By understanding how to recognize and treat infections and illnesses without relying on modern medicine, you can dramatically increase your chances of surviving during a crisis. Proper hygiene, nutrition, hydration, and access to basic herbal remedies are essential components of survival care, and these skills are crucial in any emergency. As you continue to build your survival medical knowledge, the more prepared you will be for any medical challenges that come your way. In the next chapter, we will look at environmental emergencies, including how to treat heat-related injuries, frostbite, and animal bites in survival settings.

Chapter 4: Environmental Emergencies and Health

In any survival situation, the environment poses its own set of challenges and dangers that can be just as deadly as the physical injuries or illnesses you might face. The natural world is full of hazards extreme temperatures, dangerous animals, poisonous plants, and more that require a thorough understanding of how to respond effectively. In this chapter, we'll cover how to handle a range of environmental health emergencies, from heat exhaustion to frostbite, animal bites, and poisonous plants, to ensure that you're equipped with the knowledge you need to stay safe and healthy.

Treating Heat-Related Illnesses: Heat Exhaustion vs. Heat Stroke

Heat-related illnesses are a leading cause of injury and death in outdoor survival situations, particularly during the summer months or in hot climates. When the body is unable to cool itself effectively, it can lead to a range of problems, from **heat exhaustion** to **heat stroke** both of which can have serious or even fatal consequences if not treated properly.

- **Heat Exhaustion**Heat exhaustion occurs when the body loses too much water and salt due to excessive sweating, which can impair its ability to regulate temperature. This condition is typically caused by prolonged exposure to high temperatures, especially when combined with physical exertion.
- **Symptoms of Heat Exhaustion**:

- Heavy sweating
- Weakness or fatigue
- Dizziness or lightheadedness
- Nausea or vomiting
- Headache
- Muscle cramps
- Pale, cool, or moist skin
- Rapid heart rate
- **First Aid for Heat Exhaustion**:
- **Move to a cool area**: Get the affected person into the shade or indoors to a cooler environment. If indoors, ensure the area is well-ventilated.
- **Rehydrate**: Give the person plenty of water or an electrolyte solution (preferably not caffeinated or alcoholic beverages, as they can dehydrate the body). Have them drink small sips, as large amounts of liquid at once can lead to vomiting.
- **Cool the body**: Apply cool, damp cloths to the forehead, neck, and armpits, or have the person soak in cool (but not ice-cold) water to lower their body temperature gradually. You can also fan them to aid in evaporative cooling.
- **Rest**: Ensure the person rests and remains as still as possible to avoid exacerbating the symptoms.

If the symptoms persist or worsen, heat exhaustion can progress into **heat stroke**, which is a medical emergency requiring immediate intervention.

- **Heat Stroke**Heat stroke is a far more serious condition that occurs when the body's temperature regulation system fails entirely, and the body's temperature rises above 104°F (40°C). This leads to the breakdown of critical bodily systems and can result in organ failure, brain damage, or death if not treated quickly.
- **Symptoms of Heat Stroke**:
- High body temperature (104°F or higher)
- Skin that is hot, dry, and red (absence of sweating)

- Confusion, agitation, or delirium
- Rapid, shallow breathing
- Rapid heart rate or irregular heartbeat
- Loss of consciousness
- Seizures
- **First Aid for Heat Stroke**:
- **Call for emergency help**: Heat stroke is a medical emergency that requires immediate medical attention. If possible, call for help or transport the person to the nearest healthcare facility.
- **Cool the body quickly**: Move the person into the shade or a cool environment immediately. Begin cooling efforts by applying cold compresses to the body, focusing on areas like the neck, armpits, groin, and wrists.
- **Hydrate**: If the person is conscious and able to swallow, give them small sips of cool water or an electrolyte solution. Avoid giving them cold water too quickly, as it could cause nausea or vomiting.
- **Immerse in cold water**: If available, submerge the person in a cold-water bath, or use ice packs wrapped in towels. Immersing the individual in cool water or ice will help bring the core temperature down rapidly.
- **Monitor**: Keep the person under constant observation. Be aware that in severe cases, they may lose consciousness and require CPR or other advanced medical interventions.

It's critical to understand that **prevention** of heat-related illnesses is often more effective than treatment. Always stay hydrated, wear loose-fitting, light-colored clothing, and avoid overexertion in extreme heat. It's important to take breaks regularly and never underestimate the risks of dehydration.

Cold-Weather Injuries: Hypothermia and Frostbite

In cold weather or harsh winter conditions, cold-related injuries like **hypothermia** and **frostbite** are serious concerns. When the body is exposed to extreme cold for prolonged periods, it can lose heat faster than it can produce it, leading to dangerous drops in body temperature and frostbite, especially in extremities.

- **Hypothermia**Hypothermia occurs when the body's temperature falls below 95°F (35°C). It can happen in temperatures as high as 50°F (10°C) if a person is wet and exposed to wind. The body becomes unable to generate enough heat to maintain a normal temperature, and its core systems begin to shut down.
- **Symptoms of Hypothermia**:
- Shivering (initially)
- Slurred speech or confusion
- Clumsiness or difficulty walking
- Numbness or loss of coordination
- Slow, weak pulse and breathing
- Pale or blue-tinged skin
- Loss of consciousness (in severe cases)
- **First Aid for Hypothermia**:
- **Get the person out of the cold**: Move the individual into a warmer environment as soon as possible, or shelter them from the wind if you're still outdoors.
- **Remove wet clothing**: Wet clothing draws heat away from the body. Replace it with dry, insulated clothing or blankets to retain warmth.
- **Gradually warm the body**: Begin warming the person with blankets, sleeping bags, or by sharing body heat. Use warm (but not hot) compresses on areas like the chest, armpits, and groin, where blood vessels are closer to the skin's surface.
- **Hydrate**: If the person is conscious and alert, give them warm, non-alcoholic, non-caffeinated drinks. Avoid giving them hot drinks immediately, as this could cause burns or shock.
- **Avoid rapid warming**: Do not attempt to warm the person with hot water or a heating pad, as it can cause shock and further damage. Similarly, avoid massaging the limbs, as this can lead to tissue damage.
- **Monitor closely**: Continue to monitor their body temperature and keep them as still as possible. In severe cases, you may need to seek medical

attention immediately.

Preventing hypothermia is about dressing in layers, staying dry, and avoiding exposure to wet and windy conditions. Always keep extra clothing and emergency shelters in your survival kit, particularly when traveling in cold environments.

- **Frostbite**Frostbite occurs when skin and underlying tissues freeze due to prolonged exposure to extremely cold temperatures. The most commonly affected areas are the fingers, toes, ears, and nose.
- **Symptoms of Frostbite**:
- Skin appears pale, gray, or blue
- Skin feels hard or waxy to the touch
- Numbness or a tingling sensation
- Swelling or blisters (in severe cases)
- **First Aid for Frostbite**:
- **Get to warmth**: Bring the person into a warm shelter immediately to prevent further tissue damage.
- **Warm the affected area**: Gradually warm the frostbitten skin by soaking it in warm (not hot) water (98-104°F / 37-40°C). Alternatively, warm the affected areas with body heat (e.g., placing hands under armpits or placing frostbitten toes on a warm part of the body).
- **Don't rub**: Never rub or massage the frostbitten areas, as this can cause further damage to tissues. Additionally, don't use direct heat, like heating pads, as this can burn the skin.
- **Protect the affected areas**: After warming, gently cover the affected areas with clean, loose bandages or gauze to avoid further injury.
- **Avoid walking on frostbitten feet or toes**: If the feet or toes are affected, avoid putting weight on them until they have been treated.

Frostbite prevention involves wearing proper clothing, including **insulated gloves, socks, and boots**, and avoiding prolonged exposure to extreme cold or wet conditions. Always be mindful of **wind chill**, which can accelerate frostbite.

Preventing and Treating Frostbite in Survival Settings

In a survival scenario, especially when you're stuck in the wilderness or caught in severe winter conditions, you'll need to have a set of strategies for protecting yourself and others from frostbite.

1. **Proper Clothing**: Layers are key to staying warm. Always dress in **moisture-wicking base layers**, followed by **insulated** and **windproof outer layers**. Avoid wearing tight clothing, as it restricts circulation.
2. **Regular Breaks**: Stop to take shelter and warm up at regular intervals to avoid prolonged exposure to the elements. If hiking or traveling in cold environments, plan frequent rest breaks in a shelter or insulated area.
3. **Proper Nutrition and Hydration**: Eating high-calorie, energy-dense foods helps the body generate heat. Keep a stock of food that provides **complex carbohydrates** and **healthy fats**, as well as hot drinks that provide comfort and hydration.

Managing Hypothermia: Signs, Symptoms, and First Aid

In extreme cold, hypothermia is a real threat, and survival situations that lead to prolonged exposure to the elements make this particularly dangerous. It is essential to recognize the early warning signs and take steps to rewarm the body and seek help as quickly as possible.

- **Stages of Hypothermia**:

1. **Mild Hypothermia (90-95°F / 32-35°C)**: Shivering, confusion, and slurred speech.
2. **Moderate Hypothermia (82-90°F / 28-32°C)**: Increased confusion, slurred speech, loss of coordination.
3. **Severe Hypothermia (below 82°F / 28°C)**: Shivering stops, uncon-

sciousness, and organ failure.

If you suspect severe hypothermia, emergency medical intervention is required. However, early and moderate hypothermia can be managed with **gradual rewarming** and **hydration** until professional medical care is available.

By understanding how to treat environmental injuries like heat-related illnesses, frostbite, hypothermia, and how to manage dehydration and exposure, you're significantly improving your chances of survival in extreme conditions. Always be prepared for the environment you're in whether it's the blistering heat of a desert or the bone-chilling cold of winter. Adaptation, prevention, and quick action are critical components of managing these emergencies in survival situations.

In the next chapter, we'll focus on how to handle animal bites and stings, including how to deal with venomous bites, insects, and wild animal attacks in survival settings.

Chapter 5: Dealing with Chronic Conditions in an Emergency

In survival situations, the ability to manage chronic conditions such as diabetes, hypertension, asthma, and heart disease becomes even more critical. These conditions often require consistent medication and monitoring, which may be impossible to access when traditional healthcare systems are disrupted. Understanding how to manage these chronic health issues in an emergency, along with strategies for improvising care when necessary, is crucial for maintaining health and ensuring survival. In this chapter, we'll explore practical approaches for dealing with chronic conditions when help is not available, with a focus on common conditions such as diabetes, heart disease, asthma, and epilepsy.

Managing Diabetes in Survival Situations

Diabetes is a metabolic disorder that affects the body's ability to produce or use insulin, leading to high blood sugar (hyperglycemia) or low blood sugar (hypoglycemia). Both conditions can be life-threatening if not managed properly. In a survival situation, where access to insulin, glucose testing devices, and medical supervision is limited, people with diabetes must rely on their knowledge of the disease and make adjustments to maintain their health.

- **Symptoms of Hypoglycemia (Low Blood Sugar)**:
- Sweating

- Shaking
- Irritability or confusion
- Dizziness or lightheadedness
- Rapid heartbeat
- Headache
- Weakness or fatigue
- **Symptoms of Hyperglycemia (High Blood Sugar)**:
- Frequent urination
- Increased thirst
- Dry mouth
- Fatigue or drowsiness
- Blurred vision
- Nausea or vomiting
- **Managing Hypoglycemia**:Low blood sugar is a serious condition that can quickly lead to unconsciousness or seizures if not addressed. In a survival scenario, you may not have immediate access to glucose tablets or syrups, so improvisation is important.
- **Immediate Treatment**: If someone with diabetes shows signs of hypoglycemia, the first step is to provide a fast-acting carbohydrate. This could be in the form of fruit juice, regular soda (not diet), or honey. In a pinch, any source of sugar will help raise their blood glucose levels quickly.
- **Rest and Monitoring**: After administering sugar, encourage the person to sit or lie down and rest while their blood sugar stabilizes. Keep monitoring for signs of recovery, which should happen within 10-15 minutes.
- **Food Intake**: Once the immediate symptoms are alleviated, follow up with a balanced meal that contains carbohydrates and protein to stabilize blood sugar levels over time. This can include nuts, bread, or other stable food items.
- **Managing Hyperglycemia**:If a person with diabetes is experiencing high blood sugar, the primary treatment is hydration. High blood sugar can lead to dehydration, so encourage the individual to drink plenty of

water. However, it's important to note that treating hyperglycemia in a survival setting without insulin can be challenging.

- **Hydration**: Water will help flush out excess glucose through urine. The person should be encouraged to drink small sips of water every 10-15 minutes, avoiding sugary drinks that could exacerbate the problem.
- **Physical Activity**: Moderate physical activity can help lower blood sugar by improving insulin sensitivity. If safe and feasible, have the person take a light walk or do mild exercises to reduce their blood sugar level.
- **Monitor for Complications**: Without access to insulin, prolonged hyperglycemia can lead to diabetic ketoacidosis (DKA), a life-threatening condition. Signs of DKA include fruity-smelling breath, nausea, vomiting, and confusion. Immediate medical care is necessary if DKA develops.
- **Preparing for a Survival Situation with Diabetes**:Those with diabetes should ensure that they are fully stocked with essential medications like insulin, syringes, and glucose monitoring supplies. If access to these supplies is impossible, understanding how to adjust diet and activity levels to manage blood sugar can be crucial. Carry a first aid kit with glucose gel, glucose tablets, or sugar, and consider training others in your group to help manage diabetes during an emergency.

Coping with Heart Conditions and Hypertension

Heart disease and hypertension (high blood pressure) are among the most common chronic conditions worldwide. Both conditions can become much more dangerous in a survival scenario, where stress, poor nutrition, and limited access to medications can exacerbate symptoms. Understanding how to manage heart disease and high blood pressure is essential for preventing complications and keeping the individual stable.

- **Signs of a Heart Attack**:
- Chest pain or discomfort
- Pain radiating to the arm, neck, back, or jaw
- Shortness of breath

- Cold sweat or nausea
- Lightheadedness or fainting
- **Managing a Heart Attack in a Survival Setting**:If someone is experiencing a heart attack, quick action is critical. While immediate access to medical care may not be possible, you can still provide life-saving first aid:

1. **Call for Help**: If possible, get the person to medical help immediately.
2. **Chew Aspirin**: If the person is conscious and not allergic to aspirin, have them chew one adult-strength aspirin. This can help thin the blood and reduce the risk of further damage to the heart.
3. **Rest and Reassure**: The individual should rest in a comfortable position. If they feel faint or lightheaded, keep them lying down with their legs elevated.
4. **Monitor Vital Signs**: Keep a close eye on the person's breathing, pulse, and level of consciousness. If the person stops breathing, initiate CPR (which will be covered in Chapter 2).

- **Managing Hypertension (High Blood Pressure)**:Hypertension can lead to stroke, heart attack, and other serious complications. In a survival setting, managing high blood pressure becomes challenging due to the potential lack of medication and the added stress of the situation.
- **Calm the Person**: Stress and anxiety can worsen hypertension, so it's important to keep the person as calm and relaxed as possible. Encourage slow, deep breathing exercises to lower blood pressure.
- **Hydration**: Ensure the individual is well-hydrated, as dehydration can raise blood pressure. Drink small amounts of water throughout the day.
- **Reduce Salt Intake**: If possible, avoid consuming salty foods, as salt can exacerbate high blood pressure. Focus on providing low-sodium foods like fruits, vegetables, and lean proteins.
- **Monitor for Complications**: Watch for signs of a hypertensive crisis, such as severe headache, dizziness, chest pain, or blurred vision. If these symptoms occur, it's critical to seek medical attention.

- **Preventing Heart Problems in Survival Situations**:In a survival setting, the best way to prevent heart issues is to manage stress, stay physically active, and eat a balanced diet. If you or someone else has a heart condition, take extra precautions to avoid overexertion and ensure that proper medications are available.

Asthma and Respiratory Conditions: What to Do When Inhalers Aren't Available

Asthma is a chronic respiratory condition that causes the airways to become inflamed and narrowed, making it difficult to breathe. An asthma attack can be triggered by various factors, including allergens, cold air, physical exertion, or stress. In a survival situation, asthma attacks can become even more dangerous if the person is unable to access their inhaler or other medication.

- **Recognizing an Asthma Attack**:
- Wheezing or whistling sound while breathing
- Shortness of breath or tightness in the chest
- Increased heart rate
- Difficulty speaking or coughing
- Pale or sweaty skin
- **Managing an Asthma Attack**:
- **Calm the Person**: Anxiety can worsen asthma symptoms, so it's important to keep the person calm and reassure them. Help them to sit upright and breathe slowly.
- **Bronchodilator (If Available)**: If the person has an inhaler or bronchodilator, administer it immediately to help open the airways. If no inhaler is available, there are a few other methods you can try:
- **Breathing Exercises**: Encourage slow, controlled breathing. The person should breathe in slowly through their nose and out through their mouth, trying to relax their body and lungs.
- **Use of Steam**: If possible, bring the person into a warm, humid environment. Steamy air can help open the airways and alleviate

symptoms. Alternatively, you can make a steam inhalation by boiling water and having the person inhale the vapor (make sure the water is not too hot to avoid burns).

- **Natural Remedies**: Herbal teas, such as **ginger** or **peppermint**, may help to open airways and reduce inflammation. **Honey** is another remedy known to soothe the throat and airways.
- **Preventing Asthma Attacks in a Survival Setting**:If you or someone else has asthma, it's important to have a plan in place before an attack occurs. Always carry extra medication and an inhaler, if possible. Keep the living space free of allergens (dust, mold, smoke) and try to avoid exposure to triggers, such as cold air or strenuous activity, when the condition is not well controlled.

Understanding Epilepsy: Handling Seizures and Other Neurological Issues

Epilepsy is a neurological disorder that causes recurring seizures. Seizures can range from mild episodes of altered consciousness to full-body convulsions. In a survival situation, having a seizure can be dangerous, especially if there is no immediate medical help available.

- **Recognizing a Seizure**:
- Sudden muscle jerking or twitching
- Loss of consciousness
- Eyes rolling back or staring
- Biting of the tongue
- Uncontrolled shaking or convulsions
- **First Aid for Seizures**:
- **Stay Calm**: If someone is having a seizure, the first thing to do is stay calm and remove any potential hazards from the area. This may include sharp objects, furniture, or anything that could cause injury during the seizure.
- **Position the Person Safely**: If the person is standing, guide them to the

ground gently to avoid falls. Place a soft item, like a jacket or cloth, under their head to prevent head injury.

- **Don't Restrict Movements**: Don't try to restrain the person during a seizure. Allow their body to move freely to prevent injury.
- **Aftercare**: Once the seizure is over, help the person into a recovery position, with their head slightly tilted downward to prevent choking in case of vomiting. Stay with the person and reassure them as they regain consciousness.
- **Preventing Seizures in a Survival Setting**:Epilepsy is managed with medications, but in a survival situation, these may not be available. Encourage stress reduction, proper hydration, and regular meals to help prevent seizures. It's also important to avoid known triggers, such as fatigue, flashing lights, or dehydration.

Conclusion: Preparing for Chronic Conditions in Emergencies

Chronic health conditions require ongoing management, and when faced with a survival situation, this becomes even more challenging. However, with the right preparation, education, and strategies, individuals with chronic conditions can still manage their health effectively in an emergency. Understanding how to recognize symptoms, improvise care, and prevent complications can significantly improve outcomes and help individuals with chronic conditions remain stable during critical situations.

By developing a survival plan that includes managing chronic conditions, you not only increase your chances of survival but also enhance your ability to support those around you who may rely on you for care. In the next chapter, we will cover ***natural remedies*** *for survival medicine, focusing on how plants, herbs, and natural substances can support health when conventional medicine is unavailable.*

Chapter 6: Natural Remedies for Survival Medicine

In survival situations, where access to modern medical supplies and medications is often limited or unavailable, turning to nature's medicine cabinet plants, herbs, and natural substances becomes an essential strategy for maintaining health and treating ailments. For centuries, humans have relied on the healing properties of plants and other natural remedies to treat a wide variety of illnesses and injuries. Understanding these remedies can give you a deeper level of self-reliance and empowerment when traditional medicine is out of reach.

This chapter will delve into the various natural remedies that can be used in a survival situation, providing you with practical knowledge on how to identify, prepare, and apply these remedies. From common medicinal plants to essential oils and even kitchen staples, you will learn how to harness the power of nature to treat infections, manage pain, promote healing, and support overall well-being.

Herbal Medicine: Using Plants for Healing

Herbal medicine is a powerful tool in survival medicine, as many plants possess medicinal properties that can be used to treat a wide variety of conditions, from infections to digestive disorders, pain relief, and even stress management. Many of these herbs are readily available in the wild, though some may need to be cultivated if you're in a long-term survival situation.

- **Common Medicinal Plants and Their Uses**:

1. **Echinacea**:Echinacea is well-known for its immune-boosting properties. It's particularly useful during the onset of colds or infections, as it helps stimulate the body's immune response and can reduce the severity of symptoms.

- **Use**: Echinacea can be consumed as a tea, tincture, or even in dried form. For tea, steep 1-2 teaspoons of dried Echinacea root or leaves in hot water for about 10 minutes.
- **Applications**: Use Echinacea at the first signs of a cold or infection to help bolster your body's natural defenses.

1. **Ginger**:Ginger is widely used for its anti-inflammatory, anti-nausea, and digestive support properties. It is particularly helpful for treating nausea, motion sickness, and digestive issues, as well as reducing inflammation and promoting circulation.

- **Use**: Ginger can be made into a tea by slicing fresh ginger root and steeping it in hot water for 10 minutes. Ginger can also be chewed directly to relieve nausea or digestive upset.
- **Applications**: Ginger can also be used to treat colds, headaches, and even muscle soreness due to its anti-inflammatory effects.

1. **Lavender**:Lavender is a soothing herb with strong calming properties. It's ideal for relieving stress, anxiety, and insomnia. Lavender can also be used to treat minor burns, insect bites, and skin irritation due to its antiseptic and anti-inflammatory qualities.

- **Use**: Lavender oil can be used for aromatherapy to help alleviate stress. It can also be applied topically to the skin to treat wounds or burns by diluting it with a carrier oil, such as coconut oil.
- **Applications**: Use lavender oil in a diffuser for calming effects or rub

diluted oil onto temples to ease headache pain. It can also be added to a warm bath to promote relaxation before sleep.

1. **Peppermint**:Peppermint is often used for its digestive benefits, especially for relieving gas, bloating, and nausea. It can also help alleviate headaches and has cooling properties that can reduce fever.

- **Use**: Peppermint tea is effective for soothing digestive discomfort and relieving nausea. The oil can also be diluted and applied to the temples or neck to relieve headaches or to cool the skin in case of fever.
- **Applications**: Peppermint is a great herb to have on hand for digestive issues, nausea, or minor pain relief.

1. **Yarrow**:Yarrow is a versatile herb that has been used for centuries to treat wounds, reduce fevers, and ease menstrual cramps. It's known for its ability to help stop bleeding and promote healing.

- **Use**: To treat wounds, apply fresh or dried yarrow leaves directly to the affected area, securing them with a bandage. To make a tea, steep dried yarrow leaves in hot water for 10 minutes.
- **Applications**: Yarrow can be used to staunch blood flow in minor cuts, bruises, or abrasions. It can also be used as an anti-inflammatory for pain relief.

1. **Garlic**:Garlic is known for its powerful antimicrobial, antiviral, and antifungal properties. It is particularly useful in treating infections and boosting the immune system. It also has cardiovascular benefits, helping to reduce cholesterol and blood pressure.

- **Use**: Garlic can be consumed raw, crushed into a paste, or used in cooking. For infections, crush or chop a garlic clove and mix it with honey to create a potent antimicrobial remedy. Garlic can also be infused in olive oil to treat skin infections and wounds.

- **Applications**: Garlic can be used as a natural antibiotic to fight off bacterial and viral infections. It's also effective in treating colds, coughs, and sore throats.

Making Tinctures, Teas, and Poultices from Wild Herbs

In a survival situation, it's important to know how to prepare herbal remedies effectively. Below are some basic methods for preparing and using herbal medicine when you are in the wilderness or in an off-grid situation.

- **Tinctures**:A tincture is a concentrated extract of an herb, made by soaking the plant material (such as leaves, roots, or flowers) in alcohol (usually vodka) for several weeks. The alcohol pulls out the medicinal properties of the plant, creating a potent remedy that can be used for a variety of conditions.
- **How to Make**: Fill a glass jar halfway with the herb of your choice (e.g., Echinacea, peppermint), and then fill the jar the rest of the way with alcohol. Seal the jar and store it in a cool, dark place for 2-3 weeks, shaking it daily. After the steeping period, strain out the plant material and store the tincture in a glass bottle.
- **Use**: A typical dosage for tinctures is 20-30 drops in water, taken 2-3 times per day. Tinctures are often used for immune support, calming, and pain relief.
- **Herbal Teas**:Herbal teas are one of the easiest ways to use medicinal herbs. Simply steep the leaves, roots, or flowers of the herb in hot water to extract its beneficial properties.
- **How to Make**: Use 1-2 teaspoons of dried herbs per cup of boiling water. Cover and steep for 5-10 minutes, then strain and drink.
- **Use**: Herbal teas can be used for a variety of ailments, including digestive issues (e.g., ginger, peppermint), sleep disturbances (e.g., chamomile, lavender), or respiratory problems (e.g., elderberry, echinacea).
- **Poultices**:A poultice is a paste made from crushed or powdered herbs mixed with water or other liquids to create a thick paste. This is

applied directly to the skin for a variety of purposes, such as reducing inflammation, drawing out infection, or soothing pain.

- **How to Make**: Crush or chop fresh herbs, such as **yarrow** or **comfrey**, and mix them with warm water or a carrier oil to create a paste. Apply the poultice to the affected area and secure it with a bandage.
- **Use**: Poultices are often used for wound care, treating infections, easing muscle pain, or reducing swelling.

The Healing Power of Essential Oils in Survival Situations

Essential oils are concentrated plant extracts that have potent therapeutic properties. In a survival situation, essential oils can be used for everything from treating wounds and burns to relieving stress and aiding sleep. Because they are concentrated, a little goes a long way, making them an excellent addition to your survival medicine kit.

- **Lavender Oil**: Known for its calming and relaxing effects, lavender oil is perfect for reducing anxiety and promoting sleep. It also has antiseptic properties and can be used to treat minor burns, insect bites, and cuts.
- **Use**: Add a few drops to a diffuser for relaxation or apply diluted oil to burns and skin irritations.
- **Tea Tree Oil**: Tea tree oil is a powerful antimicrobial and antifungal agent. It can be used to treat cuts, scrapes, and infections, as well as skin conditions like acne and athlete's foot.
- **Use**: Apply a drop or two of diluted tea tree oil to the affected area. Tea tree oil can also be used in a poultice for treating abscesses or infections.
- **Peppermint Oil**: Peppermint oil is great for alleviating headaches, nausea, and digestive issues. It has cooling and soothing properties that can relieve tension and help ease digestive upset.
- **Use**: Apply diluted peppermint oil to the temples or the back of the neck to relieve headaches, or inhale the oil to alleviate nausea.
- **Eucalyptus Oil**: Eucalyptus is often used to treat respiratory issues like congestion, colds, and coughs. It has antimicrobial properties and is a

natural decongestant.

- **Use**: Add a few drops to a bowl of hot water and inhale the steam to clear sinuses. It can also be applied to the chest in diluted form to help with breathing.
- **Frankincense Oil**: Frankincense is a grounding oil known for its anti-inflammatory, antiseptic, and mood-lifting properties. It can be used to treat skin infections, inflammation, and even as an aid for meditation and mindfulness in stressful situations.
- **Use**: Diffuse frankincense for a calming effect or apply it to sore muscles and wounds for relief.

Creating Natural Remedies from Kitchen Staples

In a survival situation, the food you have available can be more than just nutrition it can also serve as medicine. Many kitchen staples have medicinal properties that can help treat a variety of common ailments.

- **Honey**: Honey is a powerful antimicrobial agent and can be used to treat minor cuts, burns, and infections. It also has soothing properties for sore throats and can help reduce coughing.
- **Use**: Apply honey directly to wounds or burns, or mix with lemon for a soothing tea for sore throats.
- **Apple Cider Vinegar**: Apple cider vinegar is known for its antimicrobial properties and can help with digestive issues, such as acid reflux, bloating, and indigestion.
- **Use**: Mix one tablespoon of apple cider vinegar in a glass of water and drink before meals to help with digestion. It can also be diluted and used as a topical antiseptic for wounds.
- **Salt**: Salt is an excellent natural disinfectant and can be used to clean wounds or as a gargle for sore throats.
- **Use**: Dissolve salt in warm water to create a saline solution for cleaning wounds or as a mouth rinse for sore throats.
- **Coconut Oil**: Coconut oil has numerous medicinal properties, including

antimicrobial, anti-inflammatory, and antioxidant effects. It can be used to moisturize skin, treat minor burns, and promote healing.

- **Use**: Apply coconut oil directly to the skin for burns, rashes, or wounds, or use it for oil pulling to improve oral hygiene.

Conclusion: Empowering Yourself with Natural Remedies

The power of nature to heal is an invaluable asset when traditional medical supplies and services are unavailable. By learning to identify and use common plants, herbs, and natural substances, you can dramatically increase your self-reliance and be prepared to handle a variety of ailments in survival situations. While these remedies may not replace the need for professional medical care in all cases, they offer a crucial backup when conventional resources are inaccessible.

In the next chapter, we will explore ***emergency dental care****, focusing on how to deal with dental pain, broken teeth, and oral infections in a survival situation, where a dentist may not be readily available.*

Chapter 7: Emergency Dental Care

In any survival situation, injuries and health problems often arise unexpectedly, and the ability to handle them with the resources at hand can mean the difference between enduring the crisis and succumbing to it. Dental problems are no exception. While dental care is often overlooked in emergency preparedness, dental pain, broken teeth, and oral infections can be incredibly debilitating. The pain can be excruciating, and without access to a dentist, even a minor issue can escalate into a major health threat.

In this chapter, we will explore how to manage common dental emergencies in a survival situation, including how to treat toothaches, broken or lost teeth, and infections. We will also discuss how to maintain oral hygiene when you don't have access to conventional dental care and what steps you can take to prevent dental problems in a survival setting.

How to Handle Toothaches in the Wilderness

A toothache in the wilderness or a survival situation is a painful and potentially serious condition. The pain can range from mild sensitivity to extreme discomfort, and if left untreated, it can lead to further complications such as infections, abscesses, and even tooth loss. While the best course of action in a survival setting would be to seek professional dental care, this is often not an option. Therefore, understanding how to manage a toothache with natural remedies and basic supplies is critical.

- **Causes of Toothaches**:
- **Tooth decay**: Cavities can cause pain when the decay reaches the nerve

inside the tooth.

- **Gum disease**: Infection or inflammation of the gums can lead to pain and swelling.
- **Tooth abscess**: An infected tooth or gum can lead to the formation of an abscess, which can be extremely painful.
- **Trauma**: Injury to the mouth or teeth can cause toothaches, often accompanied by swelling or bleeding.
- **First Aid for Toothaches**:
- **Rinse with Saltwater**: If you're experiencing a toothache, the first step is to rinse your mouth with warm saltwater to help remove any debris and reduce swelling. Dissolve one teaspoon of salt in a cup of warm water and swish it around your mouth for about 30 seconds. This can help cleanse the affected area and provide temporary relief.
- **Cold Compress**: Apply a cold compress to the outside of your cheek near the sore tooth. The cold helps reduce inflammation and numb the pain. Hold the compress on for 15-20 minutes, then remove it for 10 minutes before reapplying.
- **Clove Oil**: Clove oil is one of the most effective natural remedies for dental pain. It contains **eugenol**, a powerful numbing agent. Dab a small amount of clove oil onto a cotton ball and gently apply it to the affected area. It can temporarily numb the pain and reduce inflammation.
- **Garlic**: Garlic is known for its antimicrobial and analgesic properties. Crush a garlic clove and apply it directly to the sore tooth. The sulfur compounds in garlic can help numb the area and fight infection.
- **Peppermint Tea**: Peppermint has a mild numbing effect that can soothe a toothache. Steep a peppermint tea bag in hot water, let it cool down, and then apply it to the affected area. The cool temperature and the mild anesthetic effect can reduce discomfort.
- **Preventing Toothaches in Survival Situations**:
- **Oral Hygiene**: In a survival situation, it's important to maintain good oral hygiene to prevent toothaches. Brush your teeth with a toothbrush and toothpaste (if available), or make a paste with **baking soda** and water if traditional toothpaste isn't an option. If a toothbrush is not available,

use **chew sticks** (such as from the **miswak** tree) or **twigs** from clean trees to help remove plaque.

- **Avoid Sugary Foods**: In a survival situation, sugar can exacerbate tooth decay, so try to avoid sugary foods and drinks, especially if they're not part of your regular food supply. If you have access to honey, use it sparingly, as it can also promote tooth decay.

Dealing with Broken or Lost Teeth

In a survival scenario, losing or breaking a tooth can be especially problematic. A fractured tooth can cause pain, difficulty eating, and a heightened risk of infection. A lost tooth, on the other hand, may not be as painful initially, but it can still pose a risk for infection or difficulty eating.

- **Types of Tooth Fractures**:
- **Chipped Tooth**: A small piece of the tooth breaks off. It may not be very painful, but it could cause sensitivity.
- **Cracked Tooth**: A crack or fracture in the tooth, which can extend into the pulp, causing severe pain and a risk of infection.
- **Broken Tooth**: A larger portion of the tooth breaks off, potentially causing intense pain and exposing the inner tooth tissue to bacteria.
- **First Aid for a Broken Tooth**:
- **Clean the Area**: Rinse your mouth with warm saltwater to remove any debris and bacteria around the broken tooth.
- **Apply Cold Compress**: Use a cold compress on the outside of your cheek near the broken tooth to reduce pain and swelling.
- **Protect the Tooth**: If the broken tooth has sharp edges, use **wax**, **gum**, or even **cotton** to cover the sharp parts and prevent further damage to the soft tissues inside the mouth.
- **Temporary Filling**: If part of the tooth has broken off and you're unable to reach a dentist, you can use **temporary dental filling material** (available at many pharmacies). This can help seal the tooth and reduce pain or sensitivity until professional help is available.

- **Managing a Lost Tooth**:
- If a tooth is knocked out (and it's a permanent tooth), there may be a chance to save it if you act quickly. Find the tooth and rinse it gently with water, being careful not to damage the root. If possible, place the tooth back into its socket or store it in **milk** to keep the root alive.
- If you can't replace the tooth, keep it moist in a clean container until you can access professional care.
- **Preventing Tooth Loss**:
- Avoid hard or brittle foods, and if necessary, protect your teeth with a mouth guard during physical activities.
- Keep your mouth and teeth clean by brushing regularly, even in a survival situation. Removing plaque and bacteria reduces the risk of cavities and decay, which can weaken your teeth.

Managing Gum Infections and Abscesses

Gum infections, such as **gingivitis** or **periodontitis**, and **abscesses** can be extremely painful and dangerous in a survival setting. A gum infection occurs when bacteria accumulate along the gum line, leading to inflammation, bleeding, and pain. An abscess, a collection of pus due to bacterial infection, is even more severe and can spread if not treated properly.

- **Symptoms of Gum Infections and Abscesses**:
- Swelling, redness, or tenderness in the gums
- Pain when chewing or brushing teeth
- Bleeding gums
- A bad taste or odor in the mouth
- Fever or swelling around the face or jaw (in the case of an abscess)
- **First Aid for Gum Infections**:
- **Saltwater Rinse**: Rinse your mouth several times a day with warm saltwater to help reduce bacteria and ease inflammation. Add a teaspoon of salt to a glass of warm water and rinse for 30 seconds.
- **Garlic Paste**: Garlic has strong antibacterial and antimicrobial proper-

ties. Crush a garlic clove and mix it with a bit of salt to create a paste. Apply the paste directly to the infected gums for 5-10 minutes, then rinse your mouth with saltwater.

- **Clove Oil**: Clove oil is a powerful antiseptic and analgesic. It can be used to numb pain from an infection and help reduce swelling. Apply a few drops of clove oil to a cotton ball and place it on the infected area for temporary relief.
- **Tea Bags**: Chamomile or black tea bags can be used as a compress for gum infections. Steep a tea bag, let it cool, and then apply it to the infected area to reduce swelling and provide soothing relief.
- **First Aid for Abscesses**:
- **Warm Compress**: A warm, damp compress can help bring the abscess to a head, promoting drainage. Apply the compress to the area for 15-20 minutes, several times a day.
- **Rinse with Saltwater**: This can help reduce the spread of infection and reduce swelling. After using the compress, rinse your mouth with warm saltwater to flush out bacteria.
- **Seek Professional Care**: If an abscess is severe and does not improve with basic care, it is essential to seek professional dental care as soon as possible. In extreme cases, untreated abscesses can lead to systemic infection and sepsis.

Preventing Tooth Decay with Limited Resources

Tooth decay occurs when bacteria in the mouth produce acids that wear down the enamel of the teeth. In a survival situation, prevention is often the best form of treatment, as access to professional dental care may be impossible. Fortunately, there are a few strategies you can use to minimize the risk of tooth decay.

- **Oral Hygiene**: Even without toothpaste, brushing your teeth with a clean cloth or using a **chew stick** from trees such as **miswak** or **Salvadora persica** can help remove plaque and food debris. Twigs from other trees can also be used to gently clean the teeth.

- **Herbal Mouthwash**: If you have access to herbs like **sage**, **mint**, or **thyme**, you can brew a tea and use it as a natural mouthwash. These herbs have antimicrobial properties that help fight the bacteria that cause tooth decay.
- **Limit Sugar**: In a survival situation, foods high in sugar can contribute to tooth decay. Try to avoid eating sugary foods, as they create an environment for harmful bacteria to thrive. If you do consume sugar, rinse your mouth with water afterward.
- **Hydration**: Drinking plenty of water helps rinse away food particles and bacteria, and it keeps your mouth hydrated, which is essential for maintaining healthy gums and teeth.

Conclusion: Surviving Dental Emergencies

Dental emergencies in a survival setting can be incredibly distressing, but with the right knowledge and resourcefulness, you can manage most situations effectively. By understanding how to handle toothaches, broken teeth, gum infections, and abscesses, you can mitigate the pain and reduce the risk of serious complications. Additionally, maintaining good oral hygiene and taking preventive measures will help ensure that your teeth and gums stay healthy, even when access to conventional dental care is unavailable.

In the next chapter, we will dive into ***advanced survival medicine****, including field surgery, handling severe bleeding, and performing life-saving interventions when professional care is out of reach. Whether you find yourself in a wilderness survival situation or navigating a long-term disaster scenario, knowing how to act in an emergency can save lives and keep you functioning in even the most extreme conditions.*

Chapter 8: Advanced Survival Medicine: Field Surgery

In the harshest survival situations, professional medical care may be unavailable for days or even longer. This means that you must be prepared to handle severe injuries, trauma, and medical emergencies on your own, without access to a fully stocked hospital or a skilled surgeon. In these cases, **field surgery** the practice of performing medical procedures in non-clinical environments becomes a crucial survival skill.

Field surgery, while a complex and specialized skill, can be learned with the proper preparation, knowledge, and tools. In this chapter, we will discuss the essentials of performing field surgery, including handling severe bleeding, suturing wounds, performing emergency amputations, and dealing with life-threatening injuries in the wilderness or survival situations. We will also explore the principles of **infection control**, **sterilization**, and **pain management** in a field setting.

Basic Techniques for Wound Suturing and Stitching

One of the most critical skills in field surgery is knowing how to properly stitch or suture a wound. Suturing is necessary to close deep cuts or lacerations, especially those that involve significant blood loss, to prevent infection and promote healing. Proper suturing can prevent the wound from reopening and reduce the risk of infection, which is a significant threat in survival situations.

- **When to Suture**:You should suture a wound only if it is deep enough to require closure, or if there is excessive bleeding that cannot be controlled by direct pressure alone. If the wound is superficial (i.e., just a minor scratch or cut), suturing is unnecessary, and the wound should be cleaned, dressed, and monitored for infection.
- **How to Perform Suturing**:

1. **Sterilize the Area**: Begin by cleaning the wound and the surrounding skin with an antiseptic solution. You can use **iodine tincture** or **hydrogen peroxide** to clean the area thoroughly. Be sure to wear **sterile gloves** if possible, and ensure the tools you are using (needle, scissors, forceps) are sterile.
2. **Local Anesthesia**: In a field setting, you may not have access to traditional local anesthetics. However, **lidocaine** (if available) can be injected around the wound site to numb the area. Alternatively, natural numbing agents like **clove oil** can be applied topically to reduce pain. It's important to note that in some cases, you may need to perform the procedure without anesthesia due to limited resources.
3. **Threading the Needle**: The most common suture technique involves using a curved needle and **non-absorbable suture** material. Begin by threading the needle through the skin on one side of the wound, making sure to leave a small amount of the suture material hanging. Pull the needle through to the other side of the wound and tie a knot to secure the suture in place.
4. **Stitching the Wound**: Use simple **interrupted stitches**, where each stitch is tied separately to ensure the wound stays closed. For longer lacerations, you may need to place several stitches across the wound, ensuring that the skin edges are aligned properly. Be sure to leave a small amount of space between each stitch to avoid tissue damage.
5. **Tying the Knot**: After completing the sutures, tie a secure knot at the end of the wound to prevent the sutures from coming undone. Make sure the knot is tight, but not too tight to prevent blood flow.
6. **Aftercare**: Once the sutures are in place, clean the wound again with

an antiseptic and cover it with a sterile dressing. The wound should be checked regularly for signs of infection. In a survival situation, you will need to monitor the wound closely and change the dressing as needed.

- **Types of Sutures**:

1. **Monofilament Sutures**: These are single-strand sutures that are smooth and less likely to harbor bacteria. They are often used for external stitches in clean, non-infected wounds.
2. **Braided Sutures**: These are multi-strand sutures that are stronger but can harbor bacteria. They are best used for internal suturing or when stronger durability is needed.

Performing Emergency Surgery: When It's a Life-or-Death Situation

In survival situations, you may encounter injuries or conditions that are severe enough to require immediate surgical intervention. These injuries, such as **penetrating trauma**, **internal bleeding**, or **foreign object penetration**, can be life-threatening and require prompt action. While it's essential to understand the basics of field surgery, it's important to remember that these procedures should only be performed if absolutely necessary.

- **Emergency Surgeries You May Encounter**:

1. **Puncture Wounds and Foreign Object Removal**:If a person is impaled by a sharp object, the first decision is whether to leave the object in place or remove it. In most cases, **leave the object in place** until you can reach proper medical care. Removing it can cause severe bleeding and worsen the injury. However, if the object is causing airway obstruction or impeding vital functions, it may need to be removed.

- **How to Remove a Foreign Object**:If removal is necessary, sterilize the area, apply pressure around the object to control bleeding, and use sterile forceps or scissors to carefully cut the object away from the wound, avoiding any additional trauma to surrounding tissues. Once the object is removed, the wound should be cleaned, and **sutured** if necessary.

1. **Controlling Severe Bleeding**:Severe, uncontrolled bleeding from a large artery or vein can be fatal within minutes. To stop severe bleeding, use a **tourniquet** (if available) to cut off blood flow to the injured limb. Apply the tourniquet **2-4 inches above** the wound site and tighten it to stop the bleeding. In some cases, **hemostatic agents** (such as **QuikClot**) can be used to accelerate blood clotting.

- **Wound Packing**: If bleeding cannot be controlled with pressure, pack the wound with a sterile gauze or clean cloth. Apply direct pressure to the packing to stop the bleeding, and elevate the affected limb if possible. Keep monitoring the wound for signs of continued bleeding.

1. **Emergency Amputations**:An amputation may be necessary in the case of a **severe crush injury** where the limb is no longer viable or when a severe infection (like **gangrene**) sets in. If the wound is life-threatening and amputation is the only option to prevent death from infection or blood loss, the procedure must be done with extreme care.

- **How to Perform an Amputation**:

1. **Prepare the Area**: Sterilize the tools and the area as much as possible. Use **sharp scissors or a knife** to cut through the flesh and bone. It's crucial to act swiftly to minimize trauma.
2. **Control Bleeding**: Before performing the amputation, apply a tourniquet above the injury to stop blood flow to the limb. After the amputation, quickly apply direct pressure to control the bleeding.
3. **Protect the Stump**: Once the limb is amputated, protect the exposed tissue with a sterile dressing. Monitor for signs of shock or infection.

How to Handle Severe Bleeding: Tourniquets, Hemostatic Agents, and More

Severe bleeding is one of the most common medical emergencies in survival situations, especially following accidents, traumatic injuries, or combat scenarios. Managing severe bleeding is a priority because uncontrolled blood loss can quickly lead to shock and death.

- **Tourniquets**:A **tourniquet** is an effective tool to control severe bleeding from an extremity when direct pressure is insufficient. A **commercial tourniquet** (such as a CAT tourniquet) is ideal, but in a survival situation, you can make an improvised tourniquet using a **rope**, **belt**, or **bandage**.
- **How to Apply a Tourniquet**:

1. Apply the tourniquet **2-4 inches above** the wound, avoiding joints. Ensure it is tightly secured to stop blood flow.
2. Tighten the tourniquet until the bleeding stops. If the bleeding persists, you can apply another tourniquet above the first, or use **hemostatic gauze** to promote clotting.

- **Hemostatic Agents**:Hemostatic agents, like **QuikClot**, are materials that promote clotting and can help stop severe bleeding. These agents work by causing blood to coagulate and form a clot more quickly.
- **How to Use Hemostatic Agents**:If you have access to a hemostatic agent, place the gauze directly onto the wound. Apply firm pressure to promote clotting. These agents are especially useful for internal or deep wounds that cannot be closed with sutures.
- **Direct Pressure**:If you don't have access to a tourniquet or hemostatic agents, the best method for stopping bleeding is applying **direct pressure** to the wound. Use a clean cloth, gauze, or even your bare hands to apply steady, firm pressure to the site of the wound. If the blood soaks through, do not remove the bandage. Instead, place additional cloths on top and continue to apply pressure.

Making Use of Local Anesthetics and Pain Management

In a field surgery situation, pain management is vital, but it can be challenging without access to professional medical supplies. There are several approaches to managing pain in a survival setting, which will allow you to proceed with necessary procedures while minimizing discomfort for the patient.

- **Local Anesthetics**:
- **Lidocaine** or other local anesthetics are ideal for numbing the area before performing surgery. However, in the wilderness, these might not be available. You can use **clove oil** (as mentioned earlier) for its mild anesthetic effect.
- **Herbal Remedies**: Certain herbs, like **willow bark** (which contains salicin, a compound similar to aspirin), can help reduce pain and inflammation. It can be used as a **tea** or applied topically to the wound.
- **Pain Relief**:
- In addition to local anesthetics, you can use natural remedies like **ginger**, **turmeric**, or **peppermint** to help relieve pain and inflammation. These herbs can be used internally as teas or topically as pastes.
- **Over-the-Counter Pain Relievers**: If you have access to them, medications like **ibuprofen** or **acetaminophen** can be used to manage pain and reduce inflammation after a procedure.

Infection Control and Sterilization Without Modern Tools

One of the greatest challenges of performing field surgery is maintaining a sterile environment. Infections can quickly develop in the absence of proper sterilization, and they can lead to severe complications or death.

- **Sterilizing Instruments**:If you have access to fire, you can sterilize instruments by holding them in the flames for a few seconds. **Boiling water** is another effective method of sterilization, and it can be used to clean wounds, tools, and bandages.

- **Creating a Sterile Field**:Try to create as clean an environment as possible. Clear the area of debris and dust, and use any available clean cloths or bandages to create a sterile workspace. Even in a survival situation, minimizing contamination can significantly reduce the risk of infection.

Conclusion: Mastering Field Surgery in Survival Situations

Field surgery is not for the faint of heart it requires steady hands, quick thinking, and the ability to improvise with limited resources. While professional medical care should always be the first choice, knowing how to perform essential surgical procedures can be the difference between life and death in a crisis.

By learning how to manage severe bleeding, perform sutures, handle amputations, and control infection, you increase your ability to help yourself and others in extreme survival situations. Always remember that when performing field surgery, ***safety*** *is paramount. If you're unsure about the procedure or it's not life-threatening, it's often better to seek professional care as soon as possible.*

In the next chapter, we will dive into ***mental health and psychological first aid****, an often-overlooked but critical component of survival medicine. Emotional resilience is just as vital as physical resilience when it comes to enduring a crisis and maintaining the strength to survive.*

Chapter 9: Mental Health and Psychological First Aid

When we think of survival situations, we often focus on physical injuries, illnesses, and the immediate dangers posed by the environment. However, the mental and emotional toll that such situations can have on individuals and groups is just as important sometimes, even more so. The psychological impact of survival stressors, such as isolation, trauma, and the constant threat to safety, can undermine the ability to think clearly, make decisions, and maintain hope. Understanding how to address mental health challenges in a survival situation is a key component of long-term survival and recovery.

This chapter will explore the importance of mental health in a survival situation, the psychological effects of trauma and stress, and the concept of **Psychological First Aid (PFA)**. We will also look at how to build emotional resilience, recognize signs of psychological distress, and offer effective support to individuals facing mental health challenges during emergencies. Whether you're alone or part of a survival group, understanding the psychological aspects of survival is crucial for staying functional, maintaining a sense of hope, and supporting others in their most vulnerable moments.

Understanding the Psychological Impact of Disasters and Survival Situations

Surviving a disaster or extended emergency situation isn't just about surviving physically it's about surviving emotionally and mentally as well. The psychological impact of long-term stress, traumatic experiences, and isolation can take a serious toll, not just on individuals but also on groups.

In extreme survival situations, the human mind is put under immense stress. The threat to life, the loss of familiar surroundings, limited access to resources, and the uncertainty of the future can cause overwhelming anxiety, depression, and fear. The strain of these factors can affect decision-making, social relationships, and the ability to function effectively.

- **Acute Stress**:This is the short-term stress response to a traumatic event. It is the body's natural reaction to a threat, and it can trigger the "fight, flight, or freeze" response. In the short term, acute stress can be helpful, as it keeps you alert and responsive to danger. However, if it is prolonged, it can lead to a **stress disorder**, impairing judgment, concentration, and memory.
- **Chronic Stress**:When the stress response is activated over an extended period of time, it can have severe effects on physical and mental health. Chronic stress can contribute to **anxiety disorders**, **depression**, and **post-traumatic stress disorder (PTSD)**. Physical symptoms, such as high blood pressure, muscle tension, and a weakened immune system, can also occur.
- **Psychological Trauma**:Trauma occurs when a person is exposed to events that overwhelm their ability to cope. In a survival context, this could include witnessing death, injury, or violence; being separated from loved ones; or facing extreme hardship. The trauma can have long-lasting emotional and psychological effects, including **nightmares**, **flashbacks**, **emotional numbness**, and difficulty trusting others.
- **Coping with Isolation**:For many, the emotional impact of being isolated in a survival scenario can be just as dangerous as the physical risks. Long-term isolation can lead to **depression**, **anxiety**, and **hallucinations**. The lack of social interaction and the absence of familiar comforts can make people feel hopeless and disconnected from reality.
- **Fear of the Unknown**:The fear of an uncertain future can also lead to increased anxiety and panic. When people are unsure of their safety, their resources, or their chances of survival, it can lead to a **constant state of**

alertness, contributing to mental exhaustion and burnout.

Psychological First Aid (PFA): Providing Immediate Support

Psychological First Aid (PFA) is an evidence-based approach to providing support to individuals in the immediate aftermath of a traumatic event or disaster. The goal of PFA is to reduce stress, promote safety, and provide emotional support to individuals affected by the crisis. Unlike traditional **first aid**, which focuses on physical health, PFA addresses emotional and psychological well-being, aiming to stabilize individuals and help them begin the process of recovery.

- **Principles of Psychological First Aid**:The primary objectives of PFA are to ensure safety, calm, and reassurance while helping people regain a sense of control. It does not involve diagnosing or treating psychological disorders but focuses on practical, supportive techniques to reduce distress and build coping skills. Key principles of PFA include:

1. **Establishing Safety**:The first priority in a survival situation is ensuring that individuals are safe from immediate harm. Once physical safety is established, focus on reducing emotional distress by ensuring the environment is as calm and supportive as possible. This includes finding shelter, protecting from weather conditions, and ensuring there are no ongoing threats.
2. **Promoting Calm**:People who are stressed or anxious may need reassurance and a sense of normalcy. Offer calm, clear, and empathetic communication to help reduce panic. Speak in a steady, soothing voice, and avoid overwhelming people with too much information at once. Let them know it's normal to feel distressed after a traumatic event.
3. **Encouraging Connection**:In a survival situation, it's easy to become isolated, but human connection is crucial for mental well-being. Encourage individuals to talk about their feelings, fears, and needs. Social support whether through family, friends, or fellow survivors helps build

resilience. You can also encourage group activities, such as preparing meals or organizing tasks, to foster a sense of teamwork.

4. **Fostering Hope**:People in survival situations often struggle with hopelessness and despair. It's essential to help them identify small, achievable goals, such as gathering food, securing shelter, or completing simple tasks. Celebrating small successes helps rebuild confidence and gives people a reason to continue pushing forward. Focus on what is possible and encourage a forward-looking mindset.
5. **Practical Assistance**:PFA also involves offering practical help in meeting the basic needs of individuals, such as access to food, water, medical care, and shelter. Addressing these needs not only provides physical comfort but also reduces feelings of helplessness and stress. Being able to contribute to the survival effort can instill a sense of purpose.

- **Active Listening and Emotional Validation**:Active listening is a vital tool in providing psychological first aid. Allow individuals to express their emotions without judgment, interruptions, or invalidation. Responding with empathy helps people feel understood, reducing their emotional burden. Simple phrases like "I hear you," "That sounds incredibly hard," or "You are not alone in this" can be incredibly soothing.

Building Emotional Resilience: Strengthening the Mind

Emotional resilience refers to the ability to adapt to and bounce back from adversity, trauma, and stress. In a survival situation, resilience is key to maintaining mental clarity, making sound decisions, and staying hopeful even in the face of overwhelming challenges.

- **What Makes People Resilient?**Emotional resilience doesn't mean being invulnerable to stress or hardship. Instead, it's about how people respond to adversity. Some factors that contribute to resilience include:

1. **Optimism and Hope**: Resilient individuals tend to maintain a positive

outlook, even when things are difficult. They have the ability to focus on the future and believe that their efforts can make a difference, even in challenging times.

2. **Self-Awareness**: Resilient people are in tune with their emotions and needs. They can recognize when they are struggling and take steps to address their emotional and psychological well-being, whether through self-care, seeking support, or engaging in grounding exercises.
3. **Problem-Solving Skills**: Resilient individuals approach problems with a calm, methodical mindset. They are more likely to break down large challenges into manageable steps and focus on what can be done immediately to improve the situation.
4. **Social Support**: Having a strong social support system is critical for resilience. People who feel connected to others are more likely to cope effectively with stress and trauma. In a survival situation, working as a team and supporting each other emotionally can help maintain group morale and individual resilience.
5. **Self-Care Practices**: Resilience is also about maintaining physical health, which has a direct impact on emotional well-being. Getting enough rest, staying hydrated, eating nutritious food, and engaging in physical activity all contribute to emotional resilience.

- **Building Resilience in Others**:In a group survival situation, building resilience isn't just about focusing on individual strength it's about fostering resilience within the group. Some strategies include:

1. **Encouraging Group Cohesion**: Foster a sense of community by encouraging group cooperation, open communication, and shared responsibilities. A well-organized group can share the emotional and physical burden, making it easier to manage stress collectively.
2. **Role Modeling**: As a leader or key member of the survival group, demonstrating calmness, optimism, and proactive problem-solving can set an example for others. Your emotional resilience can help others feel more secure and capable of handling challenges.

3. **Providing Emotional and Practical Support**: Offering emotional support to others in your group can be just as important as offering physical help. Encourage those around you to express their feelings, listen attentively, and offer practical solutions to immediate problems.

Recognizing and Responding to Psychological Distress in Others

In a survival scenario, not everyone will react to stress or trauma in the same way. Some may experience immediate emotional distress, while others may suppress their emotions or even deny that they are affected. It's crucial to recognize the signs of psychological distress so that you can offer the right support and intervene before conditions worsen.

- **Signs of Psychological Distress**:
- **Acute Stress Symptoms**: These may include irritability, hypervigilance, difficulty concentrating, poor sleep, and heightened anxiety. People may have difficulty relaxing, often feeling like they are "on edge."
- **Emotional Numbing**: Some individuals may experience a loss of emotional response. They might seem indifferent or emotionally distant, a common reaction to trauma.
- **Flashbacks or Nightmares**: People who have been exposed to trauma may experience flashbacks or vivid nightmares, reliving the traumatic event. This can disrupt sleep and impair functioning.
- **Panic Attacks**: Symptoms of a panic attack include rapid heartbeat, shortness of breath, chest pain, dizziness, and a fear of losing control. These attacks can occur in response to overwhelming stress or trauma.
- **Responding to Psychological Distress**:
- **Provide Comfort and Reassurance**: Reassure the individual that their reaction is normal in the face of stress and trauma. Let them know that it's okay to feel overwhelmed and that you are there to support them.
- **Create a Safe Environment**: Make sure the person is in a safe and calming environment, free from immediate threats. This will help them regain a sense of control.

- **Allow Time and Space**: Don't force someone to talk about their emotions if they are not ready. Sometimes, the best approach is to simply offer a comforting presence and allow them time to process the situation in their own way.

Psychological First Aid for Children in Crisis

Children are particularly vulnerable in stressful or traumatic situations. Their emotional and psychological resilience is still developing, and they may not have the coping mechanisms that adults have. Therefore, when working with children in survival settings, special attention must be given to their emotional and mental well-being.

- **Signs of Psychological Distress in Children**:
- Crying, clinging to caregivers
- Fear of separation or abandonment
- Difficulty sleeping or nightmares
- Regression (e.g., bedwetting, thumb-sucking)
- Increased irritability or tantrums
- Withdrawal or disinterest in activities they once enjoyed
- **Providing Psychological First Aid to Children**:
- **Provide Physical Comfort**: Children often need to feel physically safe before they can address their emotional concerns. Hold them, reassure them, and help them feel secure.
- **Use Simple Language**: Depending on the child's age, use simple, clear language to explain what is happening and why certain steps are being taken. Let them know that it is normal to feel scared but that they are safe.
- **Create a Routine**: Maintaining a sense of normalcy through routine can be incredibly helpful for children. This might involve setting aside time for meals, play, and sleep.
- **Validate Emotions**: Acknowledge the child's feelings and let them know that it's okay to be upset or scared. Encourage them to express their

emotions in a safe, healthy way.

Conclusion: The Vital Role of Mental Health in Survival

Surviving in extreme conditions is not just about physical endurance it's about mental and emotional resilience. Psychological First Aid, emotional resilience, and coping strategies can help individuals and groups endure the trauma, stress, and challenges of survival situations. Whether you're dealing with the immediate shock of a disaster, the isolation of a long-term emergency, or the mental toll of traumatic events, knowing how to respond to psychological distress can ensure that you remain functional and supportive, both for yourself and others.

As we continue our survival journey, remember that ***mental health is just as vital as physical health*** *in any crisis. In the next chapter, we will focus on* ***survival medicine for families****, including how to develop health plans, teach children basic first aid, and manage different health needs within a family unit. The strength of a family or survival group lies not only in physical preparedness but also in emotional support and collective resilience.*

Chapter 10: Survival Medicine for Families

In any emergency or survival situation, the well-being of your family or group is paramount. While survival skills such as shelter-building, food foraging, and medical treatment are essential for individual survival, caring for multiple people especially children, elderly relatives, or people with special medical needs requires additional preparation and strategies. The ability to manage your family's health and ensure that everyone is adequately cared for can make the difference between life and death in an extended emergency.

This chapter will explore how to develop a comprehensive family health plan for emergencies, manage different health needs in a family or group setting, and teach essential first aid skills to children and other family members. We'll also discuss how to set up communication systems within your family, practice emergency drills, and address the unique medical concerns of babies, toddlers, and the elderly in survival situations.

Developing Family Health Plans for Emergencies

A family health plan is an essential part of preparedness. It ensures that each family member's health needs are addressed, and it outlines clear protocols for dealing with medical emergencies. The goal is to have a set of guidelines and resources that everyone in the family understands and can follow during a crisis.

- **Key Elements of a Family Health Plan**:

1. **Contact Information**: Make a list of emergency contacts, including doctors, nearby relatives, and emergency services. In a survival setting, this might also include local shelters or other points of contact if evacuation is necessary.
2. **Medical History**: Compile a list of each family member's medical history, including any chronic conditions (e.g., diabetes, hypertension), allergies, current medications, and immunization records. This will ensure that you can manage these conditions effectively during an emergency.
3. **Medications**: Stock up on essential medications for chronic conditions and ensure you have enough supplies to last for an extended period. If you take prescription medications, speak with your doctor about obtaining an emergency supply or an alternative solution. This can include extra insulin for diabetes, blood pressure medications, or inhalers for asthma. Don't forget over-the-counter medications such as pain relievers, antihistamines, and cold treatments.
4. **First Aid Kits**: Ensure you have a fully stocked first aid kit that caters to the needs of everyone in your family. This should include supplies for treating cuts, burns, fractures, allergic reactions, and any specific medical concerns that your family members may have. Customizing your first aid kit to meet the specific needs of children, elderly relatives, and pets will help ensure comprehensive care.
5. **Preventative Measures**: Include preventive care measures in your plan, such as ensuring everyone has access to clean water, maintaining proper hygiene, and creating an environment that minimizes the risk of infections and illnesses.
6. **Evacuation Plan**: If evacuation is necessary, have a clear, practiced plan for how to leave your home, including how to transport family members with special needs or medical conditions. This plan should include multiple routes, emergency shelters, and supplies for transportation.

- **Medical Training for All Family Members**:Everyone in the family should have a basic understanding of first aid and emergency medical procedures. Teaching simple first aid techniques like CPR, wound care, and how to recognize symptoms of a stroke, heart attack, or allergic reaction can save lives in an emergency. Hold regular training sessions for family members to practice these skills so that they become second nature when a crisis occurs.

Teaching Children Basic First Aid and Emergency Procedures

While children may not be able to handle complex medical situations, teaching them basic first aid and emergency procedures can instill confidence and self-reliance. In an emergency, children can be valuable helpers, whether it's fetching water, assisting with basic care, or calming down other family members. Teaching them how to respond to common injuries or accidents is an important part of family preparedness.

- **Basic First Aid Skills for Children**:

1. **How to Call for Help**: Teach your children how to call emergency services or contact trusted family members. Make sure they understand their address, phone number, and how to speak clearly to a dispatcher.
2. **Treating Minor Cuts and Scrapes**: Show children how to clean and dress simple wounds. You can demonstrate how to use an antiseptic wipe and apply a bandage to a small cut or scrape. They should know how to wash their hands before and after touching a wound to avoid infection.
3. **Basic Burn Care**: Teach children how to treat minor burns by running the burn under cool water and applying a clean cloth or bandage to the area. They should understand when to seek adult help if the burn appears serious.
4. **Recognizing Poisoning**: Educate children on the dangers of ingesting unfamiliar substances, whether plants, chemicals, or spoiled food. Encourage them to report any suspicious substance immediately.
5. **Dealing with Bleeding**: Show children how to use a clean cloth or

bandage to apply direct pressure to a bleeding wound. This simple skill can help in an emergency, especially if an adult is not immediately available to assist.

6. **Basic CPR**: While children may not have the strength to perform full chest compressions, they can be taught the basics of CPR, such as calling for help and performing rescue breaths.

- **Teaching Children About Psychological First Aid**:It's just as important to teach children how to respond to emotional distress as it is to teach them physical first aid. Encourage open communication and help them understand that feelings of fear, anger, or sadness are natural during emergencies. Teach children how to calm themselves through simple techniques, such as deep breathing or counting to ten, to reduce anxiety during a stressful situation.

Setting Up Family Communication Systems in a Crisis

When a disaster strikes, communication can become disrupted, especially if you're separated from your family members or in an isolated environment. Establishing a family communication plan is essential to ensuring that everyone knows how to reach one another and how to communicate in the event of a crisis.

- **Communication Plan**:

1. **Designate Emergency Contacts**: Have one or more out-of-town contacts who can serve as the central point of communication. In case of displacement, everyone can contact this person to report their status and whereabouts. This ensures that even if phone lines or local networks are down, there's someone who can help coordinate information.
2. **Establish Meeting Points**: If communication is lost or you're separated during a disaster, designate a safe meeting place for the family. This could be your home, a nearby park, or a community shelter. It's important

that everyone knows where to go to reunite if you're not together.

3. **Emergency Communication Devices**: In a survival setting, cell phones may be unreliable, so consider having **two-way radios** (walkie-talkies) or a **satellite phone** for emergency communication. These can be invaluable in areas with no cellular service, allowing you to stay in touch with your family.
4. **Signal for Help**: Teach your family how to use visual and auditory signals to indicate distress. This could be through **whistles**, **flares**, or **signal fires** to attract attention from rescuers or nearby individuals in case of separation.

- **Practice Drills**: Just as fire drills are practiced in schools, your family should regularly practice emergency communication drills. Simulate various disaster scenarios (e.g., natural disasters, vehicle accidents, fires) and practice how to communicate and reunite at designated meeting points.

Managing Multiple Family Members with Different Health Needs

In any family, there are likely to be individuals with special medical needs, including **babies**, **elderly relatives**, or those with **chronic conditions**. It's important to understand the unique care these individuals will require in a survival situation and to have a plan in place for managing their health needs.

- **Caring for Babies and Toddlers**:Babies and toddlers have special needs, especially when it comes to nutrition, hydration, and comfort. In a survival situation, managing their needs can be a challenge, but with preparation, you can provide the essential care they need.

1. **Infant Formula and Breastfeeding**: If you have an infant, ensure that you have a sufficient supply of formula and the necessary tools for feeding. If the baby is breastfeeding, ensure that the mother has access to enough water and nutrition. If formula is unavailable, you may need to

rely on **alternative methods** of feeding (such as powdered milk, goat's milk, or making your own formula).

2. **Diapers and Hygiene**: Stock up on **diapers**, **baby wipes**, and **diaper rash ointment**. In a long-term survival scenario, you may need to rely on cloth diapers and reusable wipes. It's essential to keep babies and toddlers clean to prevent infections or rashes.
3. **Sleep and Comfort**: Babies and toddlers need to sleep regularly, and maintaining a familiar sleep routine can help reduce stress. Create a safe, warm, and comfortable sleeping space for the baby, using any available blankets or makeshift bedding.
4. **Illnesses in Infants**: Be prepared to treat minor illnesses such as colic, fever, or dehydration. Keep an infant thermometer on hand, and be prepared to use **oral rehydration solutions** to prevent dehydration if the baby experiences vomiting or diarrhea.

- **Caring for the Elderly**:Older adults may have specific needs related to mobility, medications, or chronic conditions such as arthritis, diabetes, or heart disease. In a survival situation, extra care must be taken to ensure their comfort and safety.

1. **Medications**: Stock up on any medications that elderly relatives may require. Ensure that you have an emergency supply, as running out of vital medications can have serious consequences. If necessary, consult a doctor for alternatives.
2. **Mobility Aids**: If your elderly family member uses a **walker**, **cane**, or **wheelchair**, make sure that they have access to these devices in a survival situation. If mobility becomes an issue, you may need to improvise transportation methods (such as using a sled or carrying them in a backpack or stretcher).
3. **Hydration and Nutrition**: Ensure that older adults stay well-hydrated and receive proper nutrition, as dehydration and malnutrition can exacerbate underlying health conditions. Provide easy-to-digest foods and liquids to prevent complications.

4. **Monitoring Health**: Watch for signs of common issues in elderly individuals, such as **dehydration**, **low blood sugar**, and **muscle weakness**. Have a plan in place to address these issues should they arise.

First Aid for Babies and Toddlers: Special Considerations

Children under the age of five are especially vulnerable in a survival situation. They require special attention when it comes to first aid and health management, as their immune systems and bodies are still developing.

- **Managing Fever**:Children can develop high fevers quickly. It's important to monitor their temperature regularly and use **cool compresses** to bring their temperature down. If the fever is over 102°F (39°C) and doesn't respond to cooling measures, seek help immediately.
- **Choking and CPR**:Babies and toddlers are more prone to choking, especially as they begin to eat solid food. Learn how to perform **infant CPR** and **choking rescue** maneuvers. Regularly practice these skills so you can act quickly in an emergency.
- **Poisoning**:Children often put things in their mouths, so be vigilant about keeping toxic substances away from them. If a child is suspected of poisoning, identify the substance and seek help immediately. **Activated charcoal** can help absorb toxins in some cases, but this should be administered under guidance.

Conclusion: The Role of Family Health in Survival

Family health in a survival situation is more than just about physical care; it's about ***emotional support****,* ***cooperation****, and* ***planning****. By preparing your family for emergencies, educating them about health and first aid, and developing a comprehensive family health plan, you're not just ensuring their physical safety you're providing the emotional and psychological tools they need to stay resilient through challenging times.*

Surviving a disaster or emergency is difficult, but together, as a family, you can rise to the challenge. In the next chapter, we will focus on ***the psychology of survival****, discussing how to stay calm under pressure, the mental resilience required to make life-saving decisions, and how to teach others in your group to handle stress in extreme conditions. Mental and emotional strength is just as critical as physical endurance in the battle for survival.*

Chapter 11: The Psychology of Survival: Staying Calm Under Pressure

When faced with a survival situation, one of the greatest challenges isn't just managing physical injuries or environmental hazards it's maintaining a clear mind. In times of crisis, panic, fear, and uncertainty can cloud judgment, impair decision-making, and hinder one's ability to act swiftly and effectively. In survival scenarios, your ability to stay calm under pressure, make rational decisions, and keep your mental state in check can be as important as the survival skills you have at your disposal.

This chapter will explore the psychology of survival, discussing the mental resilience required to persevere during times of crisis. We will look at the role of the **survival mindset**, how to recognize and manage panic, and how to make life-saving decisions quickly and effectively. We will also discuss how to teach mental resilience to others in your group, especially in high-stress situations, and how to cultivate a positive mindset that enhances your chances of survival.

How to Stay Calm and Think Clearly During Medical Crises

In medical emergencies, the pressure to act quickly can be overwhelming. Whether you're dealing with a severe injury, a life-threatening illness, or an environmental disaster, your ability to stay calm is essential. Panic can cloud your judgment, slow down your response, and increase the risk of making mistakes.

- **The Fight, Flight, or Freeze Response**:When faced with danger or trauma, your body enters the **fight, flight, or freeze** mode an automatic stress response that is designed to prepare you to deal with immediate threats. While this can be helpful in some situations, it can also be detrimental if it leads to panic or inaction. For example, when a loved one is injured, the instinct might be to freeze and not know how to react. Alternatively, someone might react with a rush of adrenaline and try to perform complicated medical procedures they are not equipped for.
- **Recognizing Stress Responses**:A key part of managing panic is recognizing when your stress response has been triggered. Common signs of stress include rapid breathing, heart palpitations, sweating, and a racing mind. Recognizing these physical and emotional symptoms can help you control them.
- **How to Stay Calm**:
- **Focus on Breathing**: One of the easiest and most effective ways to reduce panic is to slow down your breathing. Focus on taking deep, slow breaths inhale for four seconds, hold for four seconds, exhale for four seconds. This simple breathing technique can help calm the nervous system and reestablish control over your emotions.
- **Break Down the Problem**: In times of crisis, it's easy to become overwhelmed by the situation as a whole. Instead of thinking about everything at once, focus on breaking the problem into manageable tasks. For example, if someone is injured, first focus on stopping the bleeding, then on stabilizing the victim, and only then on treating the injury. This helps you avoid getting lost in the details and maintain a clear course of action.
- **Use Visualization**: Visualizing success or envisioning yourself succeeding in handling the situation can provide clarity and focus. Mentally rehearse what you need to do, whether it's applying a bandage or administering CPR. Visualization can help your brain find calm solutions during moments of panic.
- **Positive Self-Talk**: Remind yourself that you are capable and prepared. Self-affirmation and positive self-talk can reframe your mindset from

panic to control. Telling yourself "I can do this" or "I know what I need to do" helps ground you in the moment and shifts your focus away from fear.

- **Staying Calm While Assisting Others**:If you're not the one directly impacted by an emergency, your ability to stay calm will have a powerful effect on others. Your demeanor, actions, and tone of voice can either help or hinder the emotional state of those around you. To keep others calm:
- **Lead by Example**: Stay as calm as possible yourself. The more composed you are, the more likely others will follow your lead. If you begin to panic or display anxiety, it will be contagious.
- **Offer Reassurance**: Calmly explain what is happening and what steps you're taking to resolve the situation. Give them clear instructions if they need to assist, and reassure them that they are safe.

The Role of the "Survival Mindset" in Emergencies

The **survival mindset** is a mental attitude that emphasizes resilience, adaptability, and resourcefulness. People with a strong survival mindset are able to remain calm and focused even in the most dire situations. They understand that survival isn't just about physical endurance it's about mental and emotional endurance as well.

- **Core Principles of the Survival Mindset**:

1. **Adaptability**: In a survival situation, things rarely go according to plan. To survive, you need to adapt to rapidly changing circumstances. Those who have a flexible mindset can quickly shift from one solution to another, without getting bogged down by setbacks.
2. **Self-Reliance**: The survival mindset emphasizes the importance of self-reliance. It means being prepared for any situation, whether it's having the knowledge, skills, or tools needed to survive, or having the mental fortitude to solve problems and stay positive.

3. **Decision-Making Under Pressure**: Quick and effective decision-making is critical during an emergency. Those with a survival mindset are not paralyzed by indecision they trust their instincts, act decisively, and make the best possible choice with the available information.
4. **Maintaining Hope**: Having hope in the face of adversity is essential. The survival mindset teaches that even in the most hopeless situations, there is always something you can do. Holding onto hope gives you the mental strength to keep moving forward, even when things seem bleak.
5. **Mental Toughness**: Mental toughness is the ability to withstand emotional and psychological stress. It means maintaining clarity and focus despite overwhelming adversity. Those with mental toughness are able to keep their emotions in check and stay determined to survive.

- **Building the Survival Mindset**:The survival mindset can be cultivated through training, mental exercises, and past experiences. To build a survival mindset, practice the following:

1. **Practice Stressful Situations**: Simulate stressful scenarios, like practicing first aid under pressure or navigating through a difficult terrain. The more you train in challenging conditions, the easier it will be to stay calm when faced with actual crises.
2. **Challenge Yourself**: Engage in activities that push your mental and physical limits. Whether it's through physical training or mental puzzles, regularly challenging yourself strengthens your resilience and increases your confidence in your ability to overcome obstacles.
3. **Learn from Experience**: Every survival situation, even small challenges, offers a learning opportunity. Reflect on past stressful events and ask yourself: How did I handle that situation? What worked, and what could I do better next time? Continuous learning strengthens your problem-solving skills and sharpens your survival mindset.

Recognizing and Managing Panic

Panic can be one of the greatest threats to survival. In an emergency, panic can cause irrational thinking, poor decision-making, and an inability to focus on what's important. Recognizing the signs of panic, both in yourself and others, and knowing how to manage it, is essential for survival.

- **Signs of Panic**:

1. **Rapid Breathing**: One of the first signs of panic is rapid or shallow breathing. This can lead to hyperventilation, which causes dizziness and lightheadedness.
2. **Racing Thoughts**: In moments of panic, your thoughts may race, and it becomes difficult to focus. Your mind may jump from one idea to another, preventing you from considering the situation calmly.
3. **Tension and Agitation**: Panic can cause muscle tension, restlessness, and an inability to sit still. The individual may become easily agitated, speaking rapidly or reacting in a defensive manner.
4. **Overwhelming Fear**: Panic often comes with an overwhelming sense of dread or fear, leading to the "fight, flight, or freeze" response. This intense fear may make it difficult for the person to take rational action.

- **How to Manage Panic**:

1. **Breathing Techniques**: Slow, deep breathing is the most effective way to manage panic. Instruct the person to take long, slow breaths: inhale for a count of four, hold for four seconds, and exhale for four seconds. This regulates the body's response and restores control over the situation.
2. **Grounding Techniques**: If someone is panicking, grounding them in the present moment can help them focus. Ask them to pay attention to their surroundings: "What can you see? What can you hear?" Engaging their senses brings them back to the moment and away from the overwhelming fear.
3. **Reassurance and Calm Communication**: Reassure the person that

they are safe and that the situation is under control. Use a calm, steady voice to convey your message. Offer clear instructions or actions that they can take to regain control of the situation.

4. **Distraction**: In some cases, a simple distraction can help break the cycle of panic. Redirecting attention to a task or conversation can help calm the person and refocus their energy on something productive.

Decision-Making: How to Make Life-Saving Choices Quickly

During a survival scenario, decisions often need to be made quickly, with little time for contemplation. The ability to make quick, effective decisions is one of the key components of survival. It requires both mental clarity and a structured decision-making process.

- **The OODA Loop**:One of the most effective decision-making models in survival situations is the **OODA loop** (Observe, Orient, Decide, Act). This decision-making cycle was originally developed by military strategist **John Boyd** and is particularly useful when quick decisions need to be made under pressure:

1. **Observe**: Gather information about your current environment or situation.
2. **Orient**: Analyze the situation by considering past experiences, available resources, and possible outcomes.
3. **Decide**: Make a decision based on the information at hand. Trust your instincts if you don't have all the details.
4. **Act**: Implement the decision quickly and decisively. Then, evaluate the outcome and adjust your approach if necessary.

The OODA loop allows for quick analysis and effective decision-making without getting bogged down by doubt or indecision.

- **Avoiding Decision Paralysis**:In extreme situations, the sheer weight of decision-making can lead to **decision paralysis**, where you are unable to make any choices at all. To avoid this, break down large decisions into smaller, more manageable steps. For example, instead of focusing on all the details of survival, concentrate on the most immediate needs, such as **food**, **water**, and **shelter**.

Teaching Mental Resilience to Others

If you are in a group, teaching others how to handle stress and stay calm under pressure can greatly enhance the group's chances of survival. Some people naturally have more mental resilience than others, but resilience can be cultivated through practice, education, and support.

- **Group Support**: Foster a supportive environment where everyone can share their concerns, fears, and needs. Encourage open communication and provide reassurance during difficult times.
- **Group Training**: Regularly practice stressful survival scenarios with your group. These can include mock medical emergencies, simulated natural disasters, or wilderness survival drills. By practicing under pressure, you prepare your group for the real challenges ahead.
- **Positive Reinforcement**: Encourage positive thinking and reward individuals for demonstrating mental toughness. Praise their ability to stay calm, make sound decisions, and work together as a team.

Conclusion: The Mental Edge in Survival

Survival is not just about the ability to endure physically it's about staying emotionally and mentally resilient in the face of extreme adversity. The ability to remain calm, make effective decisions under pressure, and adapt to changing circumstances can significantly improve your chances of survival.

By cultivating a ***survival mindset****, learning to manage panic, and practicing mental resilience, you can handle any crisis with clarity and confidence. Whether you are facing an injury, an environmental disaster, or the emotional toll of a* *long-term survival scenario, your ability to keep your mind strong and focused is just as crucial as the physical skills you possess.*

In the next chapter, we will discuss ***preparing for long-term disasters****, including how to stockpile essential resources, create a sustainable living situation, and ensure that you can thrive even in prolonged emergencies.*

Chapter 12: Preparing for Long-Term Disasters

In the world of survival, emergencies don't always follow the timeline we expect. Natural disasters, economic collapse, pandemics, or even large-scale social disruptions can lead to extended periods where access to basic resources, including food, water, shelter, and medical care, may be severely restricted or unavailable. This is where long-term preparedness comes into play.

Surviving a short-term crisis, like a sudden storm or a few days of power outages, is one thing. But preparing for a **long-term disaster** one that stretches over weeks, months, or even years is a far greater challenge. It requires extensive planning, resource management, and a sustainable approach to living that minimizes reliance on external systems. In this chapter, we will discuss the key components of preparing for long-term disasters, including how to **stockpile essential supplies**, **create sustainable living conditions**, **plan for long-term health and medical needs**, and **develop a community survival network**. Whether you're preparing for a **natural disaster**, **economic collapse**, or any other prolonged crisis, this chapter will equip you with the tools and knowledge to thrive.

How to Stockpile Medical Supplies for Long-Term Survival

Stockpiling medical supplies is one of the most critical aspects of long-term survival planning. When facing a prolonged disaster, having access to the necessary medications, tools, and materials to treat injuries, infections, and illnesses can be the difference between life and death. In a typical emergency, medical help may be available within hours or days, but in a long-term survival situation, you must rely on your own resources.

- **Creating a Comprehensive Medical Supply Kit**:Start by building a **long-term medical kit** that addresses both common and emergency medical needs. Your kit should contain supplies to treat everything from minor injuries to major health issues. Be sure to include:

1. **Prescription Medications**: Stockpile any essential prescription medications that your family members need. This could include **insulin**, **blood pressure medication**, **inhalers** for asthma, or **epinephrine auto-injectors** for severe allergies. If possible, get extra prescriptions or find alternative medications that can be used in place of others.
2. **Over-the-Counter Medications**: Over-the-counter (OTC) medications are invaluable in treating minor illnesses and relieving symptoms. Ensure your kit includes **pain relievers** (like **ibuprofen** or **acetaminophen**), **antihistamines**, **anti-diarrheal drugs**, **cold and flu remedies**, and **antacids**. These medications can prevent unnecessary suffering during long-term crises.
3. **First Aid Supplies**: In a survival situation, injuries are inevitable. Your first aid kit should include a variety of **bandages**, **sterile gauze**, **adhesive strips**, **medical tape**, **sterile scissors**, **forceps**, **splints**, and **tourniquets**. Be sure to have **antiseptics**, such as **iodine tincture** or **hydrogen peroxide**, to clean wounds and prevent infection.
4. **Surgical Tools**: If you're preparing for a truly long-term disaster, it's important to have **surgical instruments**. These might include **scalpels**, **needles**, **sutures**, and **hemostatic agents** (such as **QuikClot**). While these tools might not be necessary in every scenario, they can be lifesaving in situations where advanced medical care is unavailable.
5. **Medical Reference Guides**: In a survival scenario, your ability to treat injuries and illnesses will depend not just on your supplies but also on your knowledge. Have a **comprehensive medical manual** or guide,

such as **The Ultimate Survival Medicine Guide**, to help you make informed decisions in emergency situations. You can also download **first aid apps** or print out guides for common injuries and illnesses that may occur.

- **Special Medical Needs**:In a long-term disaster, certain family members may have special medical needs that require extra attention. **Elderly family members**, **infants**, and people with **chronic conditions** will need tailored care. Stockpile any specialized equipment, such as **wheelchairs**, **hearing aids**, or **oxygen tanks** (if needed). Always ensure that any medical supplies are stored in a cool, dry, and secure place to avoid spoilage or degradation.
- **Considerations for Alternative Medications**:In a long-term disaster, prescription medications may become scarce, and in some cases, access to them may be entirely cut off. As part of your preparedness plan, research **alternative treatments** and **natural remedies** that can replace or supplement prescribed medications. For example, **herbal remedies** for pain relief, digestive issues, or mild infections can be invaluable in these situations.

How to Set Up a Sustainable Living Situation

In a long-term survival scenario, relying on external resources will not be an option. Whether you're facing a **collapsed economy**, a **pandemic**, or a **natural disaster**, setting up a self-sufficient living arrangement will be essential for survival. Sustainability involves ensuring that you can meet your basic needs (food, water, shelter) without being dependent on external systems.

- **Water Filtration and Storage**:One of the most critical aspects of sustainable living is having access to clean drinking water. Stockpile water, but also have systems in place to **filter** and **purify** water sources. Water filtration systems such as **Berkey filters** or **LifeStraw** are reliable options for ensuring clean water during an extended crisis. You can also learn how to purify water using **boiling** or **chemical disinfectants** (like iodine tablets or bleach).

In addition to filtering, consider long-term **water storage** systems. You can use large containers or barrels to store water, ensuring that you have access to a water supply that will last you throughout the crisis.

- **Food Storage and Preservation**:A key part of long-term survival is ensuring you have a steady and reliable food supply. Stockpiling non-perishable foods such as **canned goods**, **dried beans**, **rice**, **pasta**, **dehydrated meals**, and **freeze-dried foods** is essential. You'll need a variety of high-calorie, nutrient-dense foods to keep you energized and healthy.
- **Food Preservation Techniques**: In addition to stockpiling, you can develop sustainable methods for preserving food, such as **canning**, **fermenting**, and **dehydrating** your own produce. Growing your own **vegetables**, **herbs**, and **fruits** will also make you more self-sufficient, reducing your reliance on store-bought supplies.
- **Hunting and Fishing**: If you're in a rural area or near a body of water, hunting and fishing can provide fresh food. Learn basic **hunting** and **fishing techniques** and ensure you have the necessary tools, such as **fishing rods**, **nets**, and **traps**, as well as **knowledge of local wildlife**.
- **Shelter**:Creating a long-term shelter is a vital part of preparing for prolonged survival. If you live in an area prone to extreme weather (such as hurricanes, snowstorms, or extreme heat), you need to ensure your shelter is well-insulated, secure, and able to protect you from the elements.
- **Insulation**: Use materials like **insulating foam**, **blankets**, or **tarps** to make your shelter more comfortable and weather-resistant. If you're building a long-term shelter, consider structures like **earth berm homes**, **log cabins**, or even **tiny houses** that can be constructed with available resources.

- **Heating and Cooling**: In long-term emergencies, conventional heating or cooling systems may not be functional. You'll need to rely on alternative heat sources, such as **wood stoves**, **solar ovens**, or **camping stoves**. Ensure you have a stockpile of fuel, such as **wood**, **propane**, or **charcoal**, depending on your heat source.
- **Alternative Energy**:Powering your shelter and providing basic electrical needs will be a challenge in a long-term survival scenario. Investing in **solar panels**, **wind turbines**, or **bicycle-powered generators** can help provide sustainable energy for essential devices like communication tools, water filtration systems, or medical equipment. **Backup batteries** and **solar-powered chargers** are essential for keeping lights, radios, and other electronics running when the grid is down.

Setting Up a Long-Term Health Care System

Long-term survival will require an ongoing approach to health care. It's not enough to simply stockpile medications health maintenance and emergency care will become a daily responsibility. Preventive care, emergency protocols, and regular health monitoring should all be part of your long-term survival plan.

- **Preventive Care**:Practice good hygiene and sanitation to prevent diseases. Learn how to **sterilize equipment**, clean wounds properly, and keep your living space free from pests and pathogens. Without access to a hospital, even small infections can escalate, so being proactive about cleanliness is critical.
- **Regular Exercise**: In a survival setting, maintaining physical fitness will help you cope with the demands of daily tasks. Build a simple exercise routine to keep your body in peak condition. This will help improve cardiovascular health, strength, and endurance, which are all critical for surviving long-term.
- **Health Monitoring**:Regularly monitor the health of all family members to ensure early detection of illnesses. Keep track of vital health indicators,

such as **blood pressure**, **blood sugar**, and **weight**. Learn basic diagnostic techniques for common conditions (e.g., checking pulse, recognizing symptoms of infection, etc.) to identify problems early.

- **Managing Chronic Conditions**:In a long-term survival situation, managing chronic conditions without access to professional care can be challenging. Stockpile medications, and if necessary, seek out natural or alternative treatments to manage these conditions. Build up a robust plan for managing issues like **diabetes**, **asthma**, **heart disease**, and **high blood pressure**.

Developing a Survival Community Network

Surviving on your own can be daunting, especially in the long term. A **survival community network** is essential for building resilience, sharing resources, and ensuring that people have the support they need. Whether it's through a **neighborhood network**, **communal gardens**, or **group defense**, the power of community can make survival more manageable and even provide a sense of normalcy and hope during difficult times.

- **How to Build a Survival Network**:

1. **Start Locally**: Reach out to neighbors, local community groups, or fellow preppers to build a network of individuals you can trust in an emergency. Discuss mutual goals, resource sharing, and defense strategies.
2. **Skill Sharing**: A community is only as strong as the knowledge it possesses. Share your skills and expertise with others, whether it's **first aid**, **hunting**, **cooking**, or **building shelters**. The more skills you have within your group, the more self-reliant your community will be.
3. **Resource Pooling**: Pool resources such as food, medical supplies, and tools. This ensures that even if one family or individual faces hardship, the whole community is supported. You can also build a shared **food stockpile** and develop communal gardens for long-term sustainability.

4. **Community Defense**: In long-term survival scenarios, the threat of looters or hostile groups becomes a real concern. Develop a **community defense plan**, with clear roles, training, and protocols for ensuring the security of your group.

Conclusion: Thriving in Long-Term Survival

Preparing for long-term survival is more than just gathering supplies it's about developing a sustainable, adaptable way of life. By focusing on creating self-sufficiency in food, water, shelter, and health care, as well as building a community network for support, you can increase your chances of thriving even in the most extended disasters.

This chapter has covered essential areas of long-term survival preparedness, from stockpiling medical supplies to setting up sustainable living systems and building community networks. While no one can predict the future, by making these preparations, you will have the tools, knowledge, and mindset to face any disaster with resilience and confidence.

In the next chapter, we will look at ***the role of community in medical emergencies****, focusing on how to build an effective emergency medical team and how to share resources and knowledge within your survival network. When times are tough, community is often the most powerful resource of all.*

Chapter 13: The Role of Community in Medical Emergencies

When survival is at stake, community becomes a vital resource. In long-term survival situations, whether due to a natural disaster, economic collapse, or other large-scale emergencies, the ability to depend on others, share knowledge, and pool resources can make the difference between life and death. Medical emergencies are one area where community support becomes especially crucial. No one person can meet every medical need alone, and the strength of a survival community lies in the collective knowledge, skills, and resources that individuals bring to the table.

In this chapter, we will explore how to **build a survival medicine community**, establish **emergency medical teams**, and **share resources and medical knowledge** in a way that fosters cooperation and maximizes your group's ability to survive and thrive. By developing a medical network, you can ensure that everyone in your community has access to the care they need, especially in times when traditional healthcare systems are inaccessible.

Building a Survival Medicine Community

The foundation of a successful survival community is trust and cooperation. When medical emergencies arise, you need a network of individuals who can respond effectively, whether it's performing first aid, managing long-term health needs, or organizing care for those who are seriously injured or ill.

- **Recruiting and Identifying Key Members**:The first step in building a survival medicine community is identifying people with relevant medical knowledge and skills. While not everyone needs to be a trained medical professional, it's helpful to have a diverse group with varying expertise, including:

1. **Medical Professionals**: Doctors, nurses, paramedics, and other healthcare providers are invaluable in a survival setting. If you have access to people with medical training, make sure to include them in your network. Even if they aren't formally trained, individuals with extensive first aid knowledge or experience in emergency medical situations can be incredibly useful.
2. **First Aid and CPR Trainers**: While advanced medical knowledge is important, everyone in the community should have a basic understanding of first aid and CPR. These skills can save lives in the early stages of an emergency. If you don't have healthcare professionals, look for individuals who are trained in first aid, emergency response, or CPR.
3. **Herbalists and Alternative Medicine Practitioners**: In the absence of pharmaceuticals or modern medicine, **herbal remedies** and **alternative treatments** can play an important role. If you have someone in your community knowledgeable about herbal medicine, they can help manage minor illnesses, infections, and other health issues using natural remedies.
4. **Logistics and Support Personnel**: A survival community needs more than just medical personnel. People with organizational skills, the ability to secure and distribute supplies, and leadership experience are crucial in ensuring that medical care is provided in an efficient and coordinated manner. Support personnel are also needed for tasks like maintaining sanitation, cooking, cleaning wounds, and creating a shelter.

- **Communication Systems**:Communication is essential for effective medical management in any community. During a crisis, especially if resources are scarce and healthcare facilities are overwhelmed, clear and effective communication ensures that everyone's needs are addressed efficiently.

1. **Establish Clear Lines of Communication**: Make sure there's a system in place for sharing critical information, especially during an emergency. This could be through radios, cell phones (if available), walkie-talkies, or even signal systems like flares or whistles in case of a communication breakdown. Set up a method to broadcast messages across the community to alert everyone about medical needs, new supplies, or dangerous conditions.
2. **Create a Medical Triage System**: In times of crisis, you may have more patients than you can treat at once. A **triage system** helps prioritize care based on the severity of the injury or illness. For example:

- **Green** (minor injuries): Can wait for treatment
- **Yellow** (serious, but not life-threatening): Needs attention soon
- **Red** (life-threatening): Requires immediate treatment
- **Black** (deceased or beyond saving): No medical intervention possible

Having a clear triage protocol will help prevent chaos and ensure that those who need immediate care are prioritized.

Establishing Emergency Medical Teams

In a survival community, medical emergencies can range from minor injuries and illnesses to life-threatening conditions. Having a designated **emergency medical team (EMT)** is vital for ensuring that there is always someone trained and ready to respond to a crisis.

- **Training Emergency Medical Teams**:

1. **Basic Medical Training**: Ensure that every member of the community has basic first aid knowledge. This includes CPR, wound care, bandaging, splinting fractures, recognizing the signs of shock, and how to manage common medical emergencies like burns, heart attacks, or allergic

reactions.

2. **Specialized Training**: Some community members should undergo more advanced training, especially if you have people with complex medical needs (e.g., diabetes, heart disease). Medical professionals can help train others in how to manage these conditions, administer medications, and provide more specialized care.
3. **Practice Regular Drills**: Just like preparing for a natural disaster, practice medical drills regularly. Simulate accidents, illnesses, and other medical emergencies, and allow the community to practice their roles. This helps build confidence, improve response times, and fine-tune your triage systems.
4. **Assign Roles and Responsibilities**: Assign specific roles to each member of the emergency medical team based on their training and skills. Some individuals might be responsible for wound care, others for administering medications, and others for managing the medical supply stockpile. Having clear roles ensures that the response to an emergency is organized and efficient.

- **Medical Leadership**:Appoint someone to oversee the health and medical needs of the entire community. This **medical leader** can make critical decisions regarding treatment plans, resources, and medical strategies. It's important that the medical leader has both knowledge and leadership skills, as their decisions will impact everyone's well-being.

Sharing Resources and Medical Knowledge

One of the key aspects of a survival medicine community is resource sharing. In a long-term survival situation, it's unlikely that any one person or family will have enough medical supplies to last indefinitely. Cooperation and resource-sharing will help everyone access the care they need.

- **Resource Pooling**:

1. **Medical Supplies**: Everyone should contribute to a communal **medical stockpile**. This includes **bandages**, **medications**, **first aid kits**, **surgical supplies**, **herbal remedies**, and anything else that might be needed. Encourage families or individuals to donate what they can and to contribute extra items whenever possible.
2. **Food and Nutrients**: Good nutrition is essential for maintaining health. Ensure that the food you store is nutrient-dense and supports overall health. Special consideration should be given to individuals with **nutritional deficiencies** or specific dietary needs (e.g., children, pregnant women, elderly individuals). Community gardens, food sharing, and even shared foraging efforts can supplement food supplies.
3. **Medical Knowledge Sharing**: Everyone in the community should have access to a shared knowledge base. If you have medical professionals or people with specialized knowledge (e.g., herbalists, physiotherapists), make sure they share their knowledge with the rest of the community. Hold regular **training sessions** where people can learn new skills, share medical knowledge, and improve their emergency response skills. Having a **community health manual** or **shared medical journals** can be helpful.
4. **Barter and Trade**: In a long-term survival scenario, trade becomes a crucial means of obtaining necessary medical supplies. If your community has a good surplus of one medical item, it can be exchanged for another resource. **Bartering systems** can help ensure that all members of the community have access to what they need, especially if traditional money is no longer viable.

Community Healing Practices and Mutual Support

Physical health is critical, but so is mental and emotional well-being, especially during long-term survival situations. A community's ability to support each other emotionally can significantly enhance overall survival chances.

- **Emotional and Psychological Support**:In a prolonged disaster, individuals are likely to experience feelings of loss, grief, trauma, and despair. The key to emotional survival is having a strong support system. Create safe spaces for people to talk about their fears and struggles, and provide emotional reassurance and comfort. Encouraging emotional resilience is as important as physical survival, as it helps individuals cope with ongoing stress and hardship.
- **Healing and Group Therapy**:Many communities in long-term survival scenarios benefit from informal group therapy sessions or shared healing practices. Group discussions, storytelling, music, and even creative arts can help people process trauma, grief, and emotional distress. These activities allow individuals to share their feelings in a supportive environment and reduce isolation.
- **Restorative Practices**: Use activities like **meditation**, **yoga**, **deep breathing exercises**, or **mindfulness** to help reduce stress and increase mental resilience. Simple practices that focus on grounding and calming the mind can help members stay mentally strong in the face of adversity.

When to Call for Help: Knowing Your Limits and Resources

While a well-prepared survival community can address most medical emergencies, there may come a point when **outside help** is required. Knowing when to seek assistance is critical in life-or-death situations. It's important to recognize your community's limitations and be realistic about what you can handle without professional medical intervention.

- **Signs That You Need Professional Help**:

1. **Severe Trauma**: Major injuries that involve **severe blood loss**, **head trauma**, or **broken bones** beyond your ability to treat may require professional care.
2. **Uncontrollable Infections**: If an infection is spreading rapidly or if **sepsis** is suspected, immediate professional intervention may be needed.

3. **Mental Health Crises**: Severe mental health issues, such as **psychosis**, **extreme depression**, or **suicidal behavior**, may require intervention from a mental health professional.

In a survival scenario, help might be a long distance away, but having a **plan for communication** and **reaching out** to outside resources (whether via satellite phone, radios, or community networks) can help connect you with the assistance you need.

Conclusion: The Power of Community in Medical Emergencies

In long-term survival situations, community becomes the cornerstone of resilience. The collective strength of a group that works together to meet everyone's physical, emotional, and psychological needs is what truly defines survival. Building a strong medical community, sharing resources, pooling knowledge, and supporting each other emotionally can significantly improve your chances of survival in a prolonged disaster.

The next chapter will focus on ***case studies and real-world applications*** *of survival medicine, exploring true stories of individuals and families who have successfully navigated medical emergencies and long-term survival situations. These stories will provide insight into practical survival strategies, lessons learned from mistakes, and the essential role that community support plays in surviving a disaster.*

CHAPTER 14: CASE STUDIES AND REAL-WORLD APPLICATIONS

In the world of survival medicine, theory and practice often diverge. While it's important to understand the technical skills and strategies for handling medical emergencies and long-term survival, it's the real-world stories the ones that come from actual survival situations that offer the greatest insight. The experiences of individuals, families, and communities who have faced disasters or extreme conditions can provide invaluable lessons, teach us what works, and warn us of the pitfalls to avoid.

In this chapter, we will explore several **true stories** of survival medicine in action. These case studies will highlight various survival scenarios, from natural disasters to man-made crises, and illustrate how effective medical interventions, resource management, and community support played crucial roles in survival. We will analyze what went right, what could have been improved, and the key takeaways that can be applied to future situations. Whether you're planning for a potential disaster or simply seeking to better understand the psychological, emotional, and physical demands of survival, these case studies will help you learn from others' experiences.

True Stories of Survival Medicine in Action

Case Study 1: The 1993 South Dakota Blizzard – Survival Amidst Extreme Weather

In December 1993, a **blizzard** struck the western United States, particularly impacting South Dakota. For those caught in the storm, it was a deadly force of nature. In particular, a group of snowmobilers found themselves stranded on the plains, with snowdrifts as high as 10 feet, temperatures plummeting to -40°F, and zero visibility. They were ill-prepared for such extreme conditions.

- **Medical Response**:The group included individuals with minor injuries, but one person, **John**, sustained a **severe frostbite** on both feet after being exposed to the cold for hours. As the storm worsened, the group realized they had to come up with a plan to save him, or risk losing him to the elements. They fashioned **improvised splints** to stabilize his frozen feet and used **hot water bottles** from their gear to gradually rewarm him.
- **Key Lessons**:
- **Prevention of Hypothermia and Frostbite**: The group learned that **proactive** preparation and awareness of the symptoms of hypothermia and frostbite could have prevented much of the suffering. They had some basic knowledge of how to treat the injuries, but they had no clear first aid kit and lacked knowledge of frostbite care beyond the basics.
- **Shelter and Group Strategy**: The group was able to shelter in place, but they quickly learned the importance of creating a more **insulated, windproof shelter** in the future. The storm's duration caught them off guard, and as a result, they lacked the proper **emergency supplies** to wait out such a dangerous situation.
- **Mental Resilience**: The group's survival wasn't just about physical resources; it was about **keeping spirits up**. Those who were able to maintain calm and **focus on the next steps** helped guide the group through the storm. Leadership and the ability to stay level-headed were as important as medical skills.

Case Study 2: The 2010 Chilean Miners' Rescue – A Triumph of Teamwork and Medical Preparedness

In 2010, 33 miners in **Chile** were trapped 2,300 feet underground in a **collapsed mine**. The incident initially seemed like an insurmountable disaster no one knew if the miners were alive or dead. After 17 days, rescuers finally made contact and discovered that the miners had survived, but were in desperate need of medical attention. For over two months, the miners had to endure extreme conditions lack of food, limited water, and dangerous psychological stress.

- **Medical Response**:The rescue operation involved **advanced medical care** that began long before the miners were brought to the surface. The miners were treated for dehydration, malnutrition, and the effects of **extreme isolation**. Psychological issues such as **anxiety**, **depression**, and **post-traumatic stress disorder (PTSD)** were also a significant concern.
- **Key Lessons**:
- **Psychological First Aid**: Medical teams did not only focus on physical health; they also provided **psychological first aid**. The isolation and uncertainty of their predicament had caused significant **mental distress**, and providing the miners with **emotional support** helped reduce panic, improve morale, and **maintain resilience**. The presence of mental health professionals was crucial in this scenario.
- **Teamwork and Communication**: The miners' ability to work together and maintain order during their isolation played a large role in their survival. Teamwork and maintaining effective communication were pivotal in making sure everyone's basic needs were met. The miners organized their resources efficiently and took turns to avoid using up everything in one go.
- **Medical Readiness**: Medical teams were prepared with **portable medical equipment** and made use of the limited supplies to stabilize the miners. They also worked with rescuers to ensure the miners were treated for **psychological trauma** as well as physical injuries upon being rescued.

Case Study 3: The 2004 Indian Ocean Tsunami – Medical Response and Community Support

One of the most devastating natural disasters in recent history, the **2004 Indian Ocean Tsunami** left millions of people affected across multiple countries. Over 230,000 people were killed, and the survivors faced monumental challenges in terms of medical care, shelter, and sanitation. Many of the affected areas were in remote locations, with roads and infrastructure completely destroyed.

- **Medical Response**:The medical teams that responded to the tsunami included **international aid organizations** and **local medical professionals**. Initial efforts focused on **search and rescue**, followed by the rapid establishment of **temporary clinics** to treat the injured. Common injuries included **broken bones**, **lacerations**, and **infected wounds**. The collapse of healthcare infrastructure led to many people being treated for **infections** and **malaria**, as water contamination became a major issue.
- **Key Lessons**:
- **Rapid Triage and Resource Management**: In such a large-scale disaster, having a **triage system** in place was crucial. With limited medical resources and a high number of injured individuals, decisions had to be made quickly about who could be treated immediately and who could wait. Medical teams had to manage resources judiciously to ensure that they could provide care to as many people as possible.
- **Sanitation and Disease Prevention**: One of the greatest health challenges after the tsunami was the threat of **waterborne diseases**. Many survivors were living in shelters with poor sanitation, which led to the rapid spread of diseases such as **cholera**, **diarrhea**, and **malaria**. International health organizations had to establish **clean water sources** and **sanitation measures** to prevent further deaths.
- **Community Healing**: Beyond physical injuries, the trauma of the tsunami left many survivors with severe emotional and psychological wounds. Survivors needed support not just from medical teams but from

community healing initiatives. Local community leaders played an essential role in offering comfort and **psychological first aid**.

What Went Right: Success Stories and Lessons Learned

While each case study presents its own challenges, they all illustrate the **importance of preparation**, **community support**, and **mental resilience**. Here are the key takeaways that apply across all the survival situations:

- **Preparation Saves Lives**: Whether it's medical supplies, basic survival knowledge, or psychological strategies, preparation is the key to survival. The better you are prepared, the more likely you are to withstand the challenges that arise. Stockpiling medical supplies, establishing emergency plans, and training your group in basic first aid and survival skills can drastically increase your chances of survival in an emergency.
- **Mental Resilience and Teamwork Are Critical**: In all three case studies, **mental resilience** played a significant role in survival. Keeping a clear head in times of crisis and focusing on maintaining group cohesion is vital. Teamwork is not just about physical tasks it's also about supporting one another emotionally. A strong sense of **community** and mutual support can carry individuals through even the most difficult situations.
- **The Role of Community and Leadership**: Leadership within the community makes a huge difference during a crisis. Whether it's a trained medical professional, an experienced survivor, or just someone with the ability to keep people calm and focused, leadership can help keep morale high and ensure that resources are distributed efficiently. Effective leadership also involves being **adaptive**, making difficult decisions when necessary, and inspiring others to take action.
- **Innovation in Resource Management**: Whether it's creating makeshift medical facilities, improvising with available supplies, or coming up with innovative solutions to long-term challenges, **resourcefulness** is essential. Being able to make use of what's available and learning to

stretch supplies is crucial to survival. In the case of the Chilean miners, their ability to ration food, organize tasks, and maintain a sense of order allowed them to survive for more than two months underground.

What Went Wrong: Mistakes and How to Avoid Them

While the case studies highlight successful survival strategies, they also offer important lessons about mistakes that were made. These mistakes could have cost lives if not for timely interventions or strong community leadership.

- **Lack of Preparation for Extended Survival**: In many cases, the individuals or groups involved were ill-prepared for the length of time they needed to survive. For example, in the 1993 South Dakota Blizzard, the snowmobilers had not stocked enough survival supplies, such as extra clothing or food. **Preparation for the worst-case scenario**, including long-term survival needs like shelter, warmth, and food, is essential.
- **Poor Communication and Coordination**: In the aftermath of large-scale disasters, communication often breaks down, leading to confusion and delays in providing aid. In the **2004 Indian Ocean tsunami**, many communities experienced difficulty coordinating rescue efforts due to **damaged infrastructure**. Having a robust **communication plan** and backup systems in place whether through radios, walkie-talkies, or other methods can greatly improve response times.
- **Ignoring Mental Health**: Psychological trauma is a **silent killer** in survival situations. In the early stages of the 2004 tsunami aftermath, there was limited attention paid to the **psychological recovery** of survivors, and this delayed their long-term healing process. Mental health must be considered alongside physical injuries in any survival situation, and it should be integrated into the planning and response efforts.

Key Takeaways from Real-Life Survival Scenarios

- **Comprehensive Preparation**: Always prepare not just for the immediate emergency, but also for the long-term survival needs of your group. This includes food, water, shelter, medical supplies, and, crucially, mental health care.
- **Community Support is Key**: The strength of a community lies in its ability to share resources, knowledge, and emotional support. Whether through teamwork, leadership, or mutual care, a strong survival community can weather the toughest storms.
- **Adaptability and Innovation**: Flexibility is vital in survival situations. The ability to adapt to changing circumstances and find creative solutions to new problems is a hallmark of successful survival.
- **Psychological Resilience is Just as Important as Physical Endurance**: Never underestimate the mental challenges of survival. Psychological preparedness and resilience will be just as crucial to your survival as physical strength and skill.

Conclusion

*The case studies presented in this chapter illustrate that survival is about much more than just physical endurance. It's about **mental toughness**, **community support**, **leadership**, and **adaptability**. By learning from the mistakes and successes of those who have faced extreme survival situations, you can better prepare yourself and your family for any crisis.*

*In the next chapter, we will wrap up our exploration of survival medicine and offer **final thoughts** on **continuing your education** in survival skills, including recommendations for further learning, useful resources, and ways to maintain and improve your preparedness over time. Survival is a journey, not a destination, and ongoing education is key to staying ready for any situation.*

Chapter 15: Continuing Your Education in Survival Medicine

Survival medicine is not a static skill set it's an ongoing journey of learning, practicing, and adapting. Just as the world around us changes, so too does the landscape of survival and preparedness. Disasters, both natural and man-made, evolve over time, and so too must our methods of preparation and response. The knowledge and skills required for survival, especially in long-term emergencies, can make the difference between life and death. Therefore, continuing your education in survival medicine is essential.

This chapter will focus on ways to **expand your knowledge**, keep up-to-date with survival medicine practices, and make sure you're always prepared to face the unexpected. Whether you're just starting out or are already well-versed in the basics, there are always new techniques, tools, and insights to learn. We'll discuss **recommended books**, **training courses**, **online resources**, and **real-life practice** strategies that will help you develop and refine your survival medicine skills.

The Power of Ongoing Learning in Survival Medicine

Survival medicine is an evolving field. New research, technological advancements, and real-world experiences continue to shape how we approach medical care in disaster scenarios. What was once cutting-edge knowledge a decade ago may now be outdated or supplemented by better methods.

- **Staying Updated with New Techniques**:Whether it's the latest in **emergency medical procedures**, **wound care**, or **mental health management** during disasters, staying current is key to ensuring you have the most effective tools at your disposal. While some survival medicine techniques have been passed down for generations, new approaches to treatment, including **non-pharmaceutical remedies**, **portable medical equipment**, and **innovative trauma care**, continue to emerge.
- **Adapting to New Challenges**:Each disaster has its own unique set of challenges. For example, managing medical care in an **urban collapse** will be very different from managing health in a **wilderness survival** scenario. By continuously learning about different survival settings, medical challenges, and the most effective responses, you increase your ability to adapt to any situation.
- **Real-World Experience**:There's no substitute for actual hands-on experience. While books, courses, and training sessions are critical, nothing can prepare you better than real-world application. Volunteering in disaster relief efforts, attending survival training camps, and even participating in simulated crisis scenarios will increase your confidence and ability to manage a crisis when it arises.

Books to Enhance Your Survival Medicine Knowledge

Books are an invaluable resource for anyone seeking to learn more about survival medicine. Below are some **must-read** books and guides that can help you expand your knowledge and refine your survival medicine skills:

1. **The Ultimate Survival Medicine Guide: Emergency Preparedness for ANY Disaster** by Joseph Alton, MD, and Amy Alton, ARNP

- This book offers comprehensive coverage of the essential topics in survival medicine, including injury treatment, first aid, disease prevention, and disaster preparedness. Written by two experienced medical professionals, this guide is a practical tool for both beginners and seasoned survivalists.

1. **When All Hell Breaks Loose: Stuff You Need to Survive When Disaster Strikes** by Cody Lundin

- This book emphasizes mental and physical survival during a crisis. Cody Lundin's focus on how to remain calm and rational during emergencies is especially useful for those looking to develop mental toughness and resilience.

1. **The Survival Medicine Handbook** by Dr. Joseph Alton and Amy Alton

- This practical manual is a complete guide for treating injuries and illnesses in survival situations. It covers everything from basic first aid to advanced field surgery techniques, making it an invaluable resource for long-term preparedness.

1. **Emergency War Surgery: The Survivalist's Medical Desk Reference** by the U.S. Department of the Army

- Used by military medics, this book is a thorough resource for dealing with combat-related trauma and medical emergencies. While it is geared toward wartime conditions, the lessons learned from military medicine are highly applicable in any disaster.

1. **The Herbal Medicine-Maker's Handbook: A Home Manual** by James Green

- A great resource for learning how to create herbal remedies for treating common illnesses and injuries. Knowing how to use **plants** for medicinal purposes is a critical skill for long-term survival in wilderness scenarios or when traditional medicine is not available.

1. **Where There Is No Doctor** by David Werner

- This book is an excellent reference for dealing with basic medical issues in isolated areas. It is particularly valuable for remote survival situations, offering detailed instructions for treating injuries, illnesses, and common health concerns without access to a doctor.

1. **The Doom and Bloom Survival Medicine Handbook** by Joseph Alton, MD, and Amy Alton, ARNP

- This survival guide provides clear, easy-to-follow advice on how to handle a wide range of medical issues, from simple cuts to complex traumas. It also includes **psychological tips** for maintaining emotional well-being during stressful situations.

Training Courses and Certifications

One of the best ways to ensure you are ready for any medical emergency is by **taking courses** that teach survival medicine and first aid. Here are some **recommended courses** and **certifications**:

- **American Red Cross First Aid and CPR Courses**The American Red Cross offers various first aid and CPR certification courses. These certifications are invaluable for anyone who may need to manage medical emergencies in a disaster situation. Training includes CPR, first aid, and advanced medical techniques such as AED use. Their **First Aid/CPR/AED** course is a great starting point for beginners.
- **Wilderness First Responder (WFR)**Offered by institutions such as **NOLS (National Outdoor Leadership School)** and **Wilderness Medical Institute**, the **Wilderness First Responder** course is one of the best options for those looking to expand their first aid knowledge for outdoor or survival scenarios. It covers emergency medical care for a variety of injuries and illnesses in remote areas where professional help

may not be available.

- **Tactical Combat Casualty Care (TCCC)**For those interested in more advanced survival medicine, the **Tactical Combat Casualty Care** course teaches how to treat life-threatening injuries in high-stress environments. Originally developed for military personnel, TCCC is a must for anyone who wants to be prepared for serious trauma in survival situations, especially in combat or disaster zones.
- **Emergency Medical Technician (EMT) Certification**If you're looking to take your medical knowledge to a professional level, becoming certified as an **EMT** is an excellent choice. EMT training provides in-depth knowledge of emergency medicine, including trauma care, respiratory management, and patient assessment. Many community colleges and medical training centers offer EMT courses, and certification is often required for working in disaster relief or emergency services.
- **Survival Medicine Training with Disaster Relief Organizations**Organizations such as **Doctors Without Borders** and **Red Cross** offer specialized training programs for individuals interested in disaster medicine and emergency medical response. These programs give you hands-on experience working in crisis environments, making them an invaluable resource for those preparing for long-term survival scenarios.

Online Resources and Communities

In today's digital age, online resources offer a wealth of information that can help you enhance your survival medicine knowledge. From instructional videos to forums where experienced survivalists share their tips, the internet provides a wealth of knowledge and support.

- **Survival Medicine Websites**:

1. **Doom and Bloom** (drbonesandnurseamy.com) – This site, run by Dr. Joseph Alton and Nurse Amy Alton, offers a comprehensive blog, articles, podcasts, and videos on survival medicine topics. The site also offers

books, including their popular **Survival Medicine Handbook**.

2. **The Survival Doctor** (thesurvivaldoctor.com) – Dr. Joseph Alton, a leading expert in survival medicine, provides a wealth of free medical advice through articles, how-to guides, and videos. This site focuses on medical issues that could arise in a survival scenario, such as treating infections or performing emergency surgery.
3. **Wilderness Medical Society** (wms.org) – This site provides resources for those who wish to pursue wilderness medicine, including educational articles, research, and access to training programs.

- **YouTube Channels**:

1. **The Urban Prepper** – This YouTube channel offers practical advice on a variety of preparedness topics, including first aid, survival medicine, and emergency kits.
2. **Dr. Bones and Nurse Amy** – A popular YouTube channel that offers survival medical advice on topics like wound care, disease prevention, and mental health strategies during long-term survival scenarios.

- **Survival Forums and Groups**:Online forums like **SurvivalistBoards.com** and **Reddit's r/survival** offer communities where individuals can share knowledge, ask questions, and get advice from experienced survivalists. You'll find everything from **first aid tutorials** to discussions on **advanced trauma care**.

Real-Life Practice: Applying Your Skills

While education is essential, the real test of your survival medicine knowledge comes when you put it into practice. Real-life practice and scenario-based training are critical in honing your skills and building your confidence.

- **Survival Simulations and Drills**:Engage in survival simulations and medical drills. These can range from simple home-based scenarios, such as practicing basic first aid or creating a mock medical emergency, to more complex simulations, like organizing a full community response to a disaster. Participate in or organize **wilderness survival camps**, where you practice living off the land, performing first aid, and treating injuries in real-time.

- **Volunteering in Medical Emergencies**:Volunteer with **disaster relief organizations** or **emergency medical teams** to gain hands-on experience in real-life emergencies. This could include working with the **American Red Cross**, helping with **medical triage** at community events, or assisting at local shelters during natural disasters.
- **Home Drills**:Regularly hold emergency medical drills with your family or group. Teach everyone to recognize common medical conditions (e.g., heart attacks, fractures, burns) and practice how to respond. Simulate crises like medical evacuations, mass casualties, or mass illnesses so that everyone is prepared when the real situation arises.

Conclusion: Lifelong Learning for Survival

Survival medicine is a lifelong journey of learning, practicing, and adapting to new challenges. By continually expanding your knowledge, practicing your skills, and engaging with your community, you will ensure that you are always ready for whatever challenges the future holds. Whether it's gaining hands-on experience, staying updated with new research, or learning from others, continuing your education in survival medicine will equip you to face any disaster with confidence, adaptability, and the knowledge needed to protect yourself and others.

The world of survival medicine is vast, and the more you learn, the more you realize there is to explore. With the tools, knowledge, and mindset discussed in this guide, you are better prepared to survive, adapt, and thrive in any emergency or disaster scenario.

Conclusion: Building a Resilient Future in Survival Medicine

Surviving in a world where disasters both natural and man-made are becoming more frequent and intense requires more than just physical preparation. **Survival medicine** is a crucial aspect of this preparation, where knowledge, skills, and community play essential roles. From **basic first aid** to advanced **field surgery**, from **mental health management** to **long-term self-sufficiency**, survival medicine encompasses a broad range of practices that can help ensure not only physical survival but also emotional and psychological resilience.

Throughout this guide, we've discussed how to prepare for medical emergencies in the most extreme of circumstances, how to manage **wounds**, **illnesses**, and **trauma**, and how to establish a solid foundation for both individual and community preparedness. As we've seen in real-life case studies and the lessons shared by survivors, the difference between life and death often comes down to the ability to act swiftly and calmly, armed with the right knowledge and tools.

Key Takeaways: The Core Principles of Survival Medicine

1. **Preparation is Paramount**: The most important principle in survival medicine is preparation. Stockpiling medical supplies, acquiring the necessary knowledge, and establishing emergency plans for yourself, your family, and your community will ensure you are ready to face any disaster that comes your way.
2. **Mental Resilience is Just as Important as Physical Health**: Survival situations are not only physically taxing but also mentally and emotionally challenging. Developing a **survival mindset** one focused on adaptability, problem-solving, and emotional resilience can make the difference between giving up and pushing through the crisis.
3. **Teamwork and Community Support are Crucial**: In times of crisis, no one can survive alone. Building a support network, whether through family, friends, or organized survival groups, enhances the chances of survival and helps share the load of care, resources, and emotional support.

4. **Continuous Learning and Practice**: Survival medicine, like any skill, requires ongoing education and practice. Regularly updating your knowledge through **books**, **training courses**, and **hands-on practice** ensures that you remain equipped to handle evolving medical challenges.
5. **Practical Application is Key**: Knowledge alone isn't enough. It's essential to test your skills through **real-world practice** whether through **medical drills**, **simulated survival scenarios**, or even volunteering in **disaster response efforts**. The more you can practice under pressure, the more confident and capable you will be in an actual emergency.

Preparing for the Future: Staying Resilient

The world is unpredictable, but one thing remains certain: **preparedness is empowering**. By investing in **survival medicine education**, **mental resilience**, and **community building**, you can significantly enhance your chances of thriving in any disaster. The skills you develop and the knowledge you acquire will not only increase your chances of survival but also enable you to help others during their moments of need.

Here's a final set of action steps to continue your journey toward becoming fully prepared for medical emergencies in any survival scenario:

1. **Create a Long-Term Survival Plan**: Update your emergency plan regularly. Consider **multiple disaster scenarios** (natural, man-made, health-related) and tailor your plans accordingly. Make sure your **family members** and **community** are all familiar with this plan.
2. **Expand Your Knowledge Base**: Read more survival books, take courses, and engage with survivalist communities. Consider attending **wilderness medicine courses** or **trauma care seminars** to improve your **field surgery** and **advanced first aid** skills. Stay current with new medical trends, tools, and techniques through online resources, workshops, and survival blogs.
3. **Practice Regularly**: Set aside time for regular drills. **First aid**, **CPR**, and **wilderness survival** exercises should become part of your routine.

Simulate real-life emergencies to test how well you respond under stress and adapt to different circumstances.

4. **Build and Maintain Relationships**: A survival community is only as strong as its members. Build relationships with other individuals who are also interested in preparedness and medicine. Strengthen bonds by participating in **group training** and sharing resources.
5. **Teach Others**: One of the best ways to solidify your own knowledge is by teaching others. Hold training sessions for your family, friends, or community members on essential survival and medical skills. Encourage them to keep learning and practicing as well.

Final Thoughts: Your Role in Survival

Survival medicine isn't just about knowing how to stop bleeding or diagnose illness it's about developing the mental, emotional, and practical tools necessary to adapt and thrive in the face of adversity. **Each skill you acquire**, **every lesson learned**, and **every preparedness step taken** builds your ability to face the future with confidence, resilience, and hope.

Whether you're a seasoned survivalist or just starting your journey into preparedness, remember that survival is a collective effort. **The skills and resources you accumulate** not only prepare you to survive but also enable you to support others, creating a stronger, more resilient community in the process. And at the heart of survival medicine, it's about caring for each other physically, emotionally, and mentally through both the good times and the tough ones.

As you continue your journey, embrace the knowledge, the challenges, and the rewards of survival medicine. Stay vigilant, stay prepared, and most importantly, stay compassionate. Because when disasters strike, it's not just about surviving it's about **thriving together**.

Resources for Further Learning: Books, Websites, and Training Courses

To ensure that you continue your survival journey, here are some excellent resources for deepening your understanding of survival medicine and emergency preparedness:

1. **Books**:

- *The Ultimate Survival Medicine Guide* by Joseph and Amy Alton
- *Wilderness Medicine* by William W. Forgey
- *Survival Medicine Handbook* by Joseph Alton, MD, and Amy Alton, ARNP

1. **Websites**:

- **Doom and Bloom** (drbonesandnurseamy.com) - Survival medicine website with articles, books, and videos.
- **The Survival Doctor** (thesurvivaldoctor.com) - Medical advice for survival situations.
- **Wilderness Medical Society** (wms.org) - Resources for wilderness and expedition medicine.

1. **Training Courses**:

- **Wilderness First Responder (WFR)** – Offered by NOLS and Wilderness Medical Institute (WMI).
- **Red Cross First Aid/CPR** – A foundation in first aid and CPR.
- **Tactical Combat Casualty Care (TCCC)** – Advanced trauma care for extreme situations.
- **EMT Training** – Become a certified emergency medical technician for advanced medical response.

1. **Online Communities**:

- **Reddit Survivalists** (r/survival) – Community-driven discussions about survival strategies and prepping.
- **Survivalist Boards** (survivalistboards.com) – A forum for discussing

survival and preparedness techniques.

The End of One Chapter, The Beginning of Another

In closing, the journey of survival and preparedness is never truly over it evolves with new challenges, knowledge, and experiences. With each lesson learned and each skill honed, you are preparing for whatever the future holds, ensuring you, your family, and your community are ready to not only survive but thrive. Keep learning, keep practicing, and above all stay resilient. The world may change, but with the right mindset and preparation, you can face whatever comes your way with confidence and strength.

9 788109 115504

Printed at Repro India Ltd.